First FRCR Anatomy

JP

D1141680

First FRCR Anatomy

Mock Papers

Matthew Budak MD
Specialty Registrar in Clinical Radiology,
Ninewells Hospital and Medical School, Dundee, UK

Magdalena Szewczyk-Bieda MD(Hons)
Specialty Registrar in Clinical Radiology,
Ninewells Hospital and Medical School, Dundee, UK

Richard White BSc(Med Sci) MBChB FRCR
Specialty Registrar in Clinical Radiology,
Ninewells Hospital and Medical School, Dundee, UK

Menelaos Philippou MBChB MRCS
Specialty Trainee in Clinical Radiology,
Edinburgh Royal Infirmary, Edinburgh, UK

Ganapathy Ananthakrishnan MRCS FRCR
Specialty Registrar in Radiology and Interventional Fellow,
Gartnavel General Hospital, Glasgow, UK

Edited by
Jamie Weir MBBS DMRD FRCP(Ed) FRANZCR(Hon) FRCR
Emeritus Professor of Radiology,
University of Aberdeen, UK

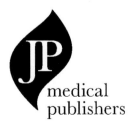

JP
medical
publishers

London • St Louis • Panama City • New Delhi

© 2013 JP Medical Ltd.
Published by JP Medical Ltd
83 Victoria Street, London, SW1H 0HW, UK
Tel: +44 (0)20 3170 8910   Fax: +44 (0)20 3008 6180
Email: info@jpmedpub.com   Web: www.jpmedpub.com

ISBN: 978-1-907816-42-0

British Library Cataloguing in Publication Data
A catalogue record for this book is available from the British Library

Library of Congress Cataloging in Publication Data
A catalog record for this book is available from the Library of Congress

JP Medical Ltd is a subsidiary of Jaypee Brothers Medical Publishers (P) Ltd, New Delhi, India

Publisher: Richard Furn
Commissioning Editor: Hannah Applin
Senior Editorial Assistant: Katrina Rimmer
Design: Designers Collective Ltd

Copy edited, typeset, printed and bound in India.

Editor's introduction

When I was approached to help in editing this text, not only was I delighted and honoured but I realised that events in radiological anatomy had come full circle. I produced my first atlas of radiological anatomy in the 1970s as a consequence of the Royal College of Radiologists' introduction of a new FRCR exam in anatomy. Its aim was to help students in their understanding of human anatomy and thus enable them to improve the care of their patients. Now Matthew Budak and his colleagues have produced this text as a result of the new format of the First FRCR exam, and it has been a pleasure to be involved with its development.

The emergence of new technology over the last 40 years has dramatically changed the way radiologists investigate patients, and the increased resolution of many techniques has lead to much greater understanding of pathology. However, in order to take full advantage of these techniques, it is imperative that 'imagers' know the fundamental appearances of normal anatomy, its variations and variants, and the subtle changes that pathology brings. Pathology is, after all, only altered anatomy and to recognise it requires knowledge of the normal!

Passing examinations is part of medical education, designed in the end to help improve the outcomes for patients, and I am convinced this text will help in that respect.

Jamie Weir
Emeritus Professor of Radiology, University of Aberdeen
Formerly both Dean and Vice-President of the Royal College of
Radiologists and Chief Examiner for the previous FRCR Part 1 exam

Preface

Although fundamental human anatomy has not significantly altered over the past century, the radiologist's ability to view and perceive the human body has been revolutionised over the last few decades. The specialty of radiology has advanced rapidly and its exponential growth has resulted in it being one of the leaders in modern day medicine. New engineering and technological feats have created an array of imaging modalities that are now seen in radiology departments around the world.

The ability to recognise the abnormal is based on the concept of being comfortable in knowing what is normal. Normal anatomy is taught on numerous occasions during different stages in our career, at medical school attending dissections or intra-operatively in surgical theatres. It is the radiologist's duty and challenge to translate this embedded knowledge and interpret both the normal and abnormal on a two-dimensional image. Through radiology training, trainees acquire the ability to read in two dimensions but see in three.

In parallel with having the fortune of cross-sectional imaging at our fingertips, comes the continual endeavour for the radiologist to further acquire the understanding of what normal looks like in great detail. Computed tomography has given us exceptional spatial resolution while magnetic resonance shows extraordinary soft tissue contrast. At times, both modalities may be utilised on any individual patient, however their portrayal of anatomy will defer. It also becomes evident that even the same modality may show great differences of how the anatomy is presented on screen, be it different contrast phases in CT or different weighted sequences in MR.

The Royal College of Radiologists re-implemented the First FRCR anatomy module in 2010. The exam focuses on normal 'radiological anatomy' utilising all current imaging modalities. The authors have reflected on their experience of the exam and have written this book to aid exam preparation. Tips and *aides-mémoires* have been included, which helped us get past this difficult yet very satisfactory hurdle in our career. The cases in this book cannot completely cover the entirety of human anatomy, however they do encompass the fundamentals of each anatomical system. Some questions will be easy whereas others will be extremely difficult.

Use this text as a start to your radiological career and continue to study normal radiological anatomy: it is fundamental to the understanding of pathology and to the expertise you bring to patients' diagnosis and treatment.

Matthew Budak
Magdalena Szewczyk-Bieda
Richard White
Menelaos Philippou
Ganapathy Ananthakrishnan
May 2012

Contents

Editor's introduction   v
Preface   vii
Exam revision advice   xi
Recommended reading   xii

Chapter 1   Mock paper 1   1

            Cases   2
            Answers   22

Chapter 2   Mock paper 2   31

            Cases   32
            Answers   52

Chapter 3   Mock paper 3   61

            Cases   62
            Answers   82

Chapter 4   Mock paper 4   93

            Cases   94
            Answers   114

Chapter 5   Mock paper 5   123

            Cases   124
            Answers   144

Chapter 6   Mock paper 6   155

            Cases   156
            Answers   176

Chapter 7   Mock paper 7   187

            Cases   188
            Answers   208

Chapter 8   Mock paper 8   217

            Cases   218
            Answers   238

Contents

Chapter 9	**Mock paper 9**	**247**
	Cases	248
	Answers	268
Chapter 10	**Mock paper 10**	**279**
	Cases	280
	Answers	300
Chapter 11	**Mock paper 11**	**309**
	Cases	310
	Answers	330
Chapter 12	**Mock paper 12**	**339**
	Cases	340
	Answers	360
Chapter 13	**Mock paper 13**	**369**
	Cases	370
	Answers	390
Chapter 14	**Mock paper 14**	**399**
	Cases	400
	Answers	420
Chapter 15	**Mock paper 15**	**429**
	Cases	430
	Answers	450
Index		**459**

Exam revision advice

At the time of publication of this book, the First FRCR anatomy module consists of 20 images, numbered 1–20. Each image has five questions labelled A–E. Candidates have 75 minutes to review all 20 images, the associated questions and record the answers on the answer sheet.

All questions are digitally presented using Osirix software running on an Apple Mac Mini workstation and displayed on a 19" monitor. To familiarise yourself with the Osirix software prior to the exam, it can be downloaded in the App stores for Macs, iPhones and iPads. Instructions on Osirix software use is provided by the examiners in a short tutorial and demo before the start of the exam. Following this tutorial, you will have the opportunity to 'test run' the software with two sample images. Once you are familiarised with the software, the exam will start.

During the exam, images may be viewed sequentially or individually. This allows candidates to return to any question at any time during the examination. All the activity of each individual workstation is centrally monitored by an invigilator.

Once the exam starts, try to remain composed during the entirety of the exam. Difficult images or questions may be presented, however try not to let this discourage you for the remainder of the exam. It is important to refrain from stalling on a single image because, from the authors' experience, there should be adequate time to return to these unanswered questions. It is important to build up confidence by answering questions which you are sure of the answer and this in turn will allow you to gain crucial marks towards your total score.

To obtain optimal marks in the exam:
- Include sides where applicable: left or right, in line with convention in cross-sectional imaging of the head, thorax and abdomen. This may be provided as a side marker on an image.
- Answer in detail, for example 'gastric fundus' is more specific than 'stomach' and '3rd part of duodenum' or 'transverse part of duodenum' is more detailed than 'duodenum' alone.
- Refrain from using abbreviations, for example write 'superior vena cava' instead of 'SVC'.
- Use all the information provided in the question booklet, for example some images may provide a brief description of the image to help orientate yourself to the anatomical system, for example 'Ultrasound of the infant hip'.
- Recall the *aides-mémoires* provided in the Answer sections of this book. These answers provide a very brief description of the pertinent anatomy that may be questioned.

This book is not intended to be a comprehensive text on radiological anatomy; instead, it allows candidates to prepare for the anatomy module with 15 mock exams, which are designed for trainees to develop knowledge, and practice and improve exam technique.

Recommended reading

Books

Weir J, Abrahams PH, Spratt JD, Salkowski LR. Imaging atlas of human anatomy (4th ed). Philadelphia: Mosby Elsevier; 2010.

Butler P, Mitchell AWM, Ellis H. Applied radiological anatomy. Cambridge: Cambridge University Press; 1999.

Ryan S, McNicholas M, Eustace SJ. Anatomy for diagnostic imaging (3rd ed). Edinburgh: Saunders; 2011.

Ahuja AT, Antonio GE. Diagnostic and surgical imaging anatomy. Ultrasound. Salt Lake City: Amirsys; 2007.

Federle MP. Diagnostic and surgical imaging anatomy. Chest, abdomen, pelvis. Salt Lake City: Amirsys; 2006.

Harnsberger HR, Macdonald AJ. Diagnostic and surgical imaging anatomy. Brain, head & neck, spine. Salt Lake City: Amirsys; 2006.

Manaster BJ. Diagnostic and surgical imaging anatomy. Musculoskeletal. Salt Lake City: Amirsys; 2006.

Manaster BJ, Crim JR, Rosenberg ZS. Diagnostic and surgical imaging anatomy. Knee, ankle, foot. Salt Lake City: Amirsys; 2007.

Online Resources

Radiographics: http://radiographics.rsna.org

radiologyanatomy.com: http://radiologyanatomy.com

IMAIOS e-anatomy: http://www.imaios.com/en

Radiologic Anatomy, Wayne State University: http://www.med.wayne.edu/diagradiology/anatomy_modules/page1.html

Radiopaedia: http://radiopaedia.org

eMedicine: http://emedicine.medscape.com

Apps

IMAIOS e-anatomy. Numerous system-based apps on subscription basis: iPhone, iPad and Android

Monster Anatomy. Individual apps for upper and lower limbs: iPhone, iPad

Chapter 1

Mock paper 1

20 cases to be answered in 75 minutes

Case 1.1

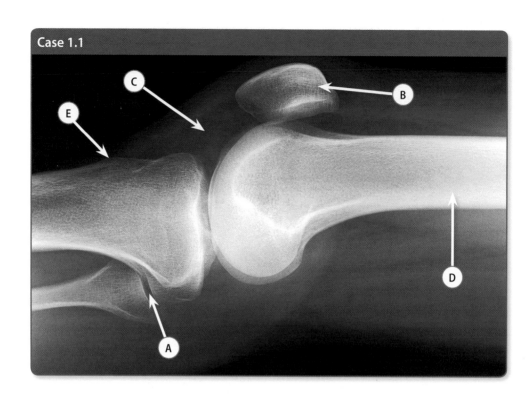

Case 1.1

QUESTION		WRITE YOUR ANSWER HERE
A	Name the structure labelled A.	
B	Name the structure labelled B.	
C	Name the structure labelled C.	
D	Name the structure labelled D.	
E	Name the structure that inserts into the structure labelled E.	

Case 1.2

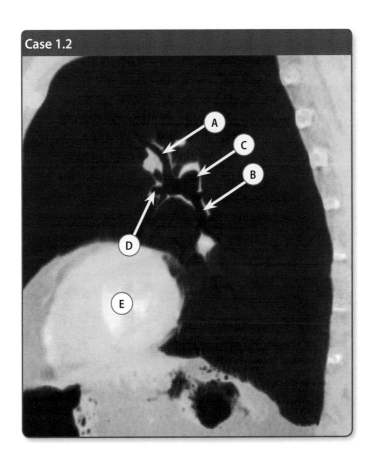

Case 1.2

QUESTION		WRITE YOUR ANSWER HERE
A	Name the structure labelled A.	
B	Name the structure labelled B.	
C	Name the structure labelled C.	
D	Name the lobar segment labelled D.	
E	Name the chamber labelled E.	

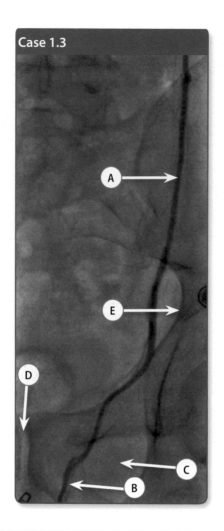

Case 1.3

Case 1.3		
QUESTION		**WRITE YOUR ANSWER HERE**
A	Name the vein labelled A.	
B	Which plexus of veins is depicted by B?	
C	Name the foramen labelled C.	
D	Name the joint labelled D.	
E	Name the osseous line labelled E.	

Case 1.4

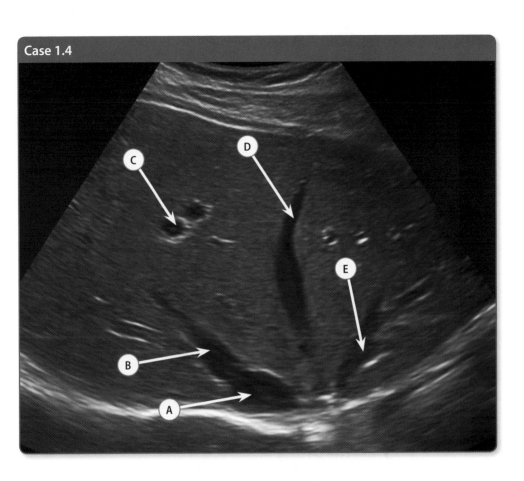

Case 1.4

QUESTION		WRITE YOUR ANSWER HERE
A	Name the structure labelled A.	
B	Name the structure labelled B.	
C	Name the structure labelled C.	
D	Name the structure labelled D.	
E	Name the structure labelled E.	

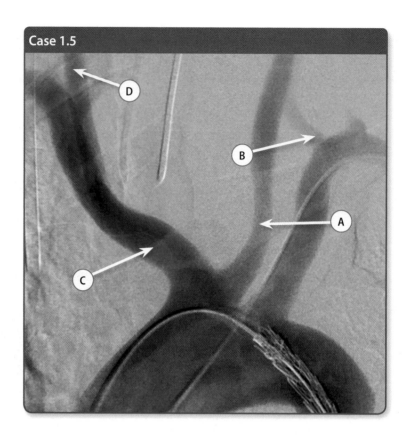

Case 1.5

Case 1.5		
QUESTION		**WRITE YOUR ANSWER HERE**
A	Name the structure labelled A.	
B	Name the structure labelled B.	
C	Name the structure labelled C.	
D	Name the structure labelled D.	
E	Which anatomical variant is present on this image?	

Case 1.6

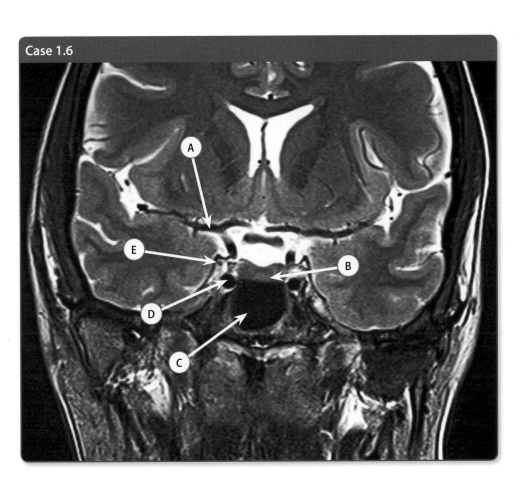

Case 1.6

QUESTION	WRITE YOUR ANSWER HERE
A Name the structure labelled A.	
B Name the structure labelled B.	
C Name the structure labelled C.	
D Name the structure labelled D.	
E Name the cranial nerve labelled E.	

Case 1.7

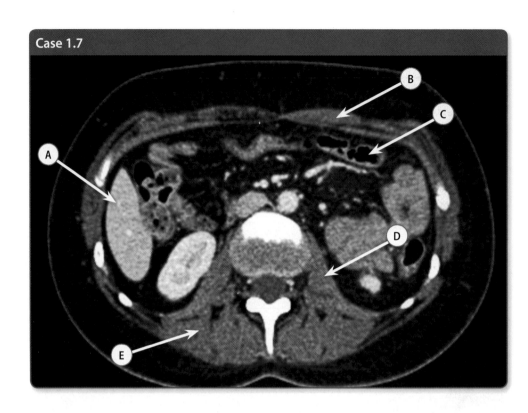

Case 1.7

QUESTION		WRITE YOUR ANSWER HERE
A	Name the structure labelled A.	
B	Name the structure labelled B.	
C	Name the colonic segment labelled C.	
D	Name the structure labelled D.	
E	Name the structure labelled E.	

Case 1.8

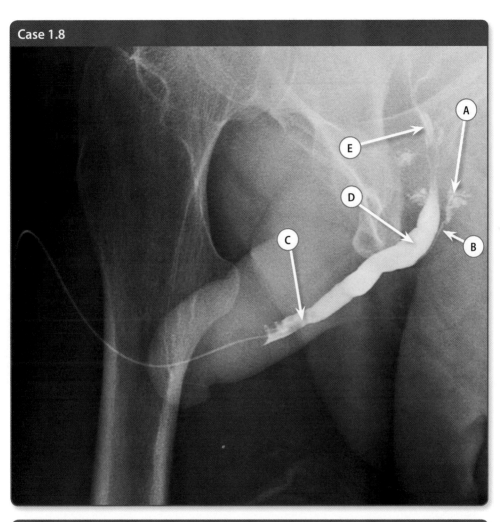

Case 1.8

QUESTION		WRITE YOUR ANSWER HERE
A	Name the structure labelled A.	
B	Name the structure labelled B.	
C	What part of the urethra does C correspond to?	
D	What part of the urethra does D correspond to?	
E	What part of the urethra does E correspond to?	

Case 1.9

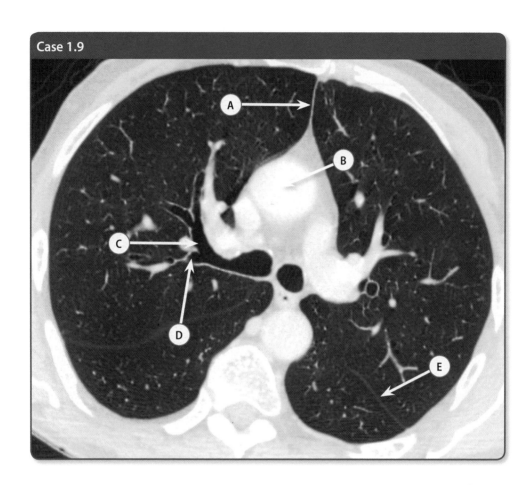

Case 1.9

QUESTION		WRITE YOUR ANSWER HERE
A	Name the structure labelled A.	
B	Name the structure labelled B.	
C	Name the structure labelled C.	
D	Name the structure labelled D.	
E	Name the linear structure labelled E.	

Case 1.10

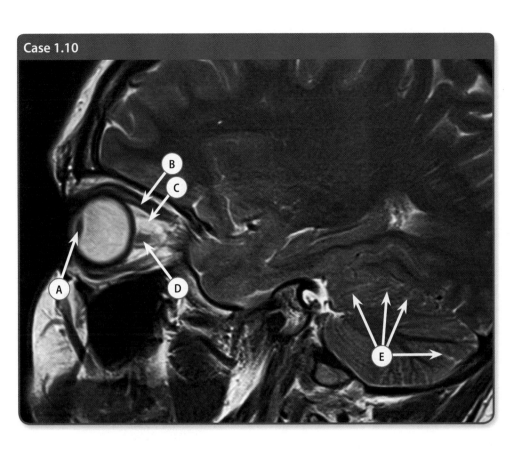

Case 1.10

QUESTION		WRITE YOUR ANSWER HERE
A	Name the structure labelled A.	
B	Name the structure labelled B.	
C	Name the structure labelled C.	
D	Name the structure labelled D.	
E	Name the spaces labelled E.	

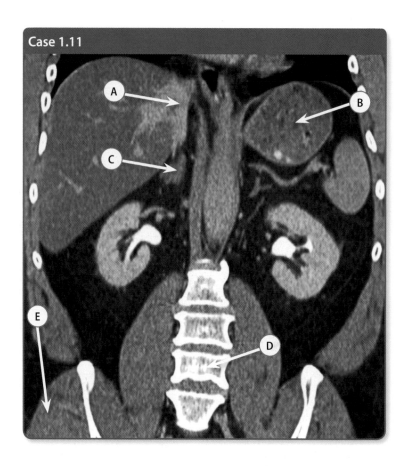

Case 1.11

Case 1.11	
QUESTION	WRITE YOUR ANSWER HERE
A Name the structure labelled A.	
B Name the structure labelled B.	
C Name the structure labelled C.	
D Name the structure labelled D.	
E Name the structure labelled E.	

Case 1.12

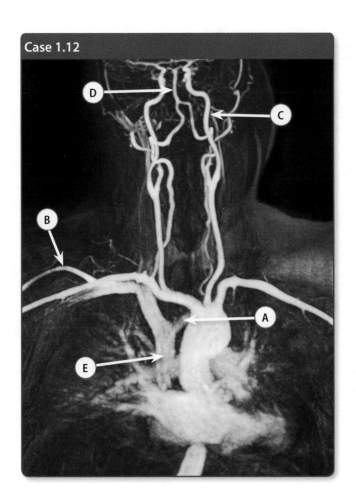

Case 1.12

QUESTION		WRITE YOUR ANSWER HERE
A	Name the structure labelled A.	
B	Name the structure labelled B.	
C	Name the structure labelled C.	
D	Name the structure labelled D.	
E	Name the structure labelled E.	

Case 1.13

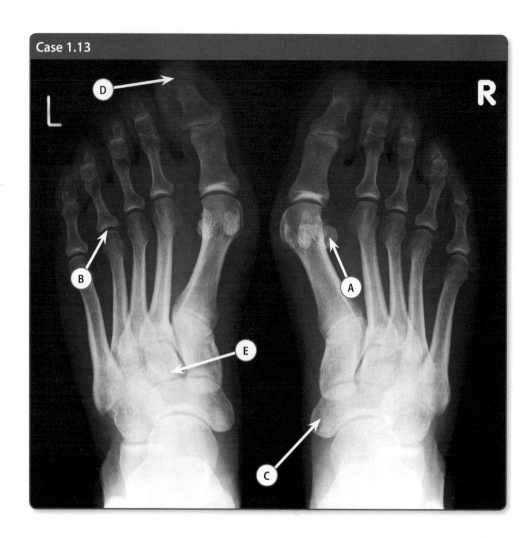

Case 1.13

QUESTION		WRITE YOUR ANSWER HERE
A	Name the structure labelled A.	
B	Name the structure labelled B.	
C	Name the structure labelled C.	
D	Name the structure labelled D.	
E	Name the structure labelled E.	

Case 1.14

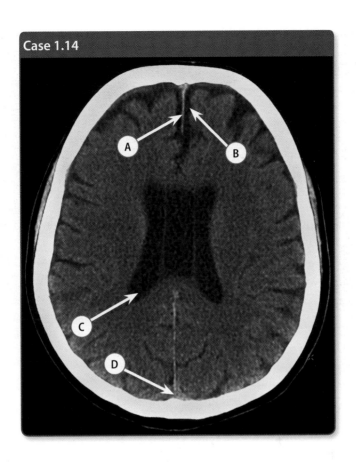

Case 1.14

QUESTION		WRITE YOUR ANSWER HERE
A	Name the structure labelled A.	
B	Name the space labelled B.	
C	Name the structure labelled C.	
D	Name the structure labelled D.	
E	Which anatomical variant is present on this image?	

Case 1.15

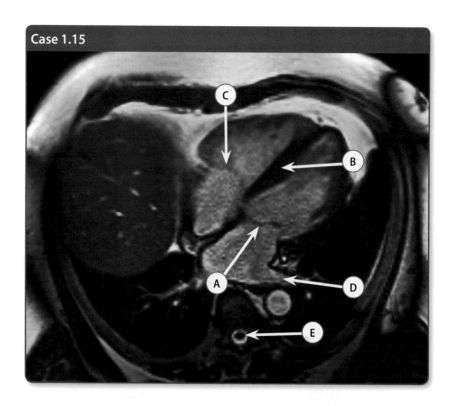

Case 1.15

QUESTION		WRITE YOUR ANSWER HERE
A	Name the structure labelled A.	
B	Name the structure labelled B.	
C	Name the structure labelled C.	
D	Name the structure labelled D.	
E	Name the structure labelled E.	

Case 1.16

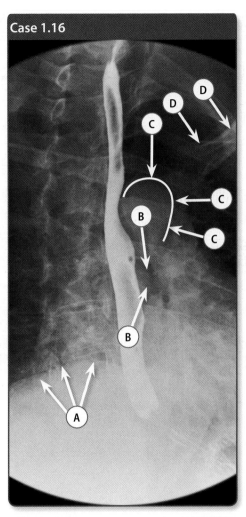

Case 1.16

QUESTION		WRITE YOUR ANSWER HERE
A	Name the structure labelled A.	
B	Name the lucent structure labelled B.	
C	Name the soft tissue density structure outlined by the arrows labelled C.	
D	Name the structure labelled D.	
E	At what vertebral level does the oesophagus normally traverse the diaphragm?	

Case 1.17

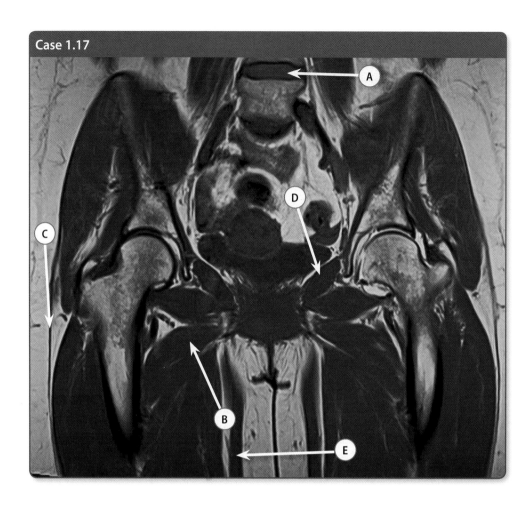

Case 1.17

QUESTION		WRITE YOUR ANSWER HERE
A	Name the structure labelled A.	
B	Name the structure labelled B.	
C	Name the structure labelled C.	
D	Name the structure labelled D.	
E	Name the structure labelled E.	

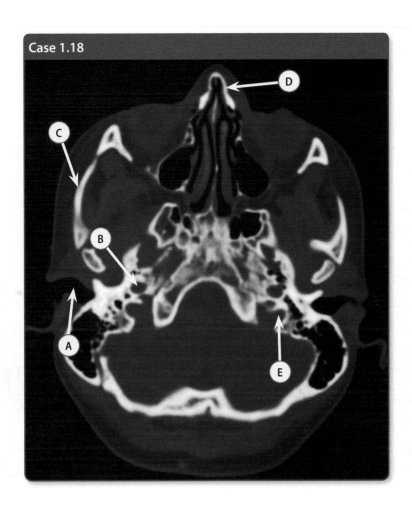

Case 1.18

	QUESTION	WRITE YOUR ANSWER HERE
A	Name the structure labelled A.	
B	Name the structure labelled B.	
C	Name the structure labelled C.	
D	Name the structure labelled D.	
E	Name the structure labelled E.	

Case 1.19

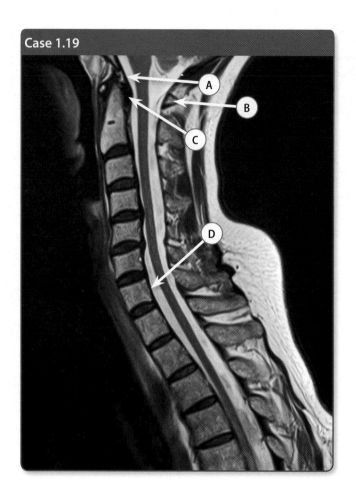

Case 1.19		
QUESTION		**WRITE YOUR ANSWER HERE**
A	Name the structure labelled A.	
B	Name the structure labelled B.	
C	Name the structure labelled C.	
D	Name the structure labelled D.	
E	What name is given to the ligament connecting the laminae of adjacent vertebrae?	

Case 1.20

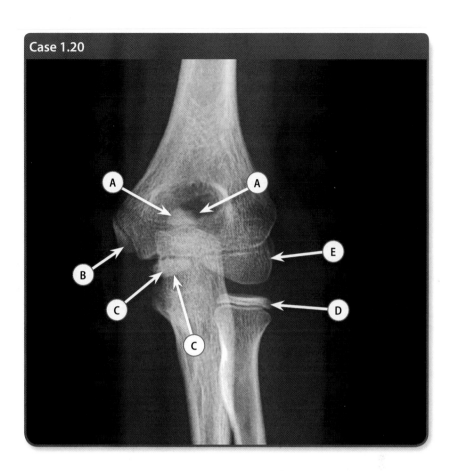

Case 1.20

QUESTION		WRITE YOUR ANSWER HERE
A	Name the ossification centre labelled A.	
B	Name the ossification centre labelled B.	
C	Name the ossification centre labelled C.	
D	Name the ossification centre labelled D.	
E	Name the ossification centre labelled E.	

Answers

Case 1.1

A Proximal tibiofibular joint

B Patella

C Infrapatellar (Hoffa's) fat pad

D Distal femoral diaphysis

E Patellar tendon

The patella lies in the anterior trochlear groove of the femur and is stabilised by the quadriceps tendon superiorly and the patellar tendon inferiorly. The patellar tendon courses superficial to Hoffa's fat pad and inserts onto the tibial tuberosity.

Case 1.2

A Apicoposterior segment bronchus of the left upper lobe

B Anteromedial basal segment of the left lower lobe

C Left lower lobe bronchus

D Superior lingular segmental bronchus

E Left ventricle

The left lung comprises two lobes, the upper and lower lobes.

The segmental anatomy of the left upper lobe includes:

- apicoposterior segment
- anterior segment
- lingula
  - superior lingular segment
  - inferior lingular segment

The segmental anatomy of the left lower lobe includes:

- superior (apical) segment
- anteromedial basal segment
- lateral basal segment
- posterior basal segment

The key to answering this question is dependent on identifying whether one is on the left or right side of the thorax. The clue lies in (E), a thick muscular walled chamber of the heart – the left ventricle.

Case 1.3

A Left testicular vein

B Left pampiniform plexus

C Left obturator foramen

D Symphysis pubis

E Left Iliopectineal line

The testicular vein drains venous blood from the pampiniform plexus of the testes. They usually drain into the left renal vein on the left and inferior vena cava on the right, but considerable variation may be seen. Understanding of venous anatomy is necessary prior to attempting embolisation for varicocoeles.

Testicular arteries are branches of the abdominal aorta arising at the level of the renal arteries.

Case 1.4

A Intrahepatic segment of inferior vena cava

B Right hepatic vein

C Branch of right portal vein

D Middle hepatic vein

E Left hepatic vein

This ultrasound image clearly shows the three hepatic veins (right, middle and left) converging to join the intrahepatic segment of the inferior vena cava, just before it drains into the right atrium. Other than different directions of flow, branches of the portal vein demonstrate increased echogenicity of the vessel wall as compared to hepatic veins.

Case 1.5

A Left common carotid artery

B Left vertebral artery

C Brachiocephalic trunk/innominate artery

D Right common carotid artery

E Common origin of left common carotid artery and brachiocephalic trunk

The second most common variant of aortic arch branching occurs when the left common carotid artery has a common origin with the innominate artery. Rather than arising directly from the aortic arch as a separate branch, the left common carotid artery origin is moved to the right and merges with the origin of the innominate artery. This variant is often termed a 'bovine aortic arch' which is a misnomer as it has no resemblance to the arterial branching pattern seen in cattle.

Case 1.6

A Right middle cerebral artery

B Pituitary gland

C Sphenoid sinus

D Cavernous portion of the right internal carotid artery

E Oculomotor nerve (CN III)

Cavernous sinuses are paired extradural venous channels situated on either side of the pituitary fossa. They communicate posteriorly with the transverse sinuses and serve as a pathway for the internal carotid artery and the III, IV, V1, V2 and VI cranial nerves.

The oculomotor nerve is the uppermost cranial nerve in the cavernous sinus, and is located lateral to the cavernous portion of the carotid artery. CN IV, V1, V2, VI lie inferior to CN III, in that order.

Case 1.7

A Right lobe of liver

B Left rectus abdominis muscle belly

C Transverse colon

D Left psoas major muscle

E Right quadratus lumborum muscle belly

The abdominal wall can be divided into three parts: anterior, lateral and posterior. Each part of the abdominal wall is comprised of multiple layers, including skin, subcutaneous fat, fascial and muscular layers and parietal peritoneum. The muscular layer of the posterior abdominal wall consists of the following muscles:

- psoas major and minor muscles medially
- quadratus lumborum and erector spinae muscles laterally
- iliacus muscle inferiorly
- diaphragm superiorly

Case 1.8

A Cowper's (bulbourethral) gland

B Duct of bulbourethral gland

C Penile urethra

D Bulbous urethra

E Prostatic urethra

Retrograde urethrography is used to demonstrate structural abnormalities of the urethra, including strictures and (in the event of trauma) urethral disruption. It is performed by placing the tip of a catheter inside the navicular fossa – a focal dilatation just proximal to the urethral meatus – and instilling contrast in a retrograde manner. Anatomically, the male urethra is divided into posterior and anterior portions. The posterior urethra comprises the prostatic urethra (the portion passing from the bladder neck through the prostate) and the membranous urethra (which extends through the urogenital diaphragm). The anterior urethra is composed of the bulbar urethra (between the urogenital diaphragm and root of the penis) and the penile urethra. The navicular fossa and meatus may also be included with the anterior urethra.

The paired Cowper's (or bulbourethral) glands are exocrine glands which are equivalent to Bartholin's glands in females.

Case 1.9

A Anterior junctional line

B Ascending aorta

C Anterior segmental bronchus of right upper lobe

D Apical segmental bronchus of right upper lobe

E Left oblique fissure

The right main bronchus divides into the right upper lobe bronchus and bronchus intermedius. The bronchus intermedius gives off the middle and lower lobe bronchi.

Case 1.10

A Lens

B Superior rectus muscle

C Retro-orbital fat

D Optic nerve

E Cerebellar folia

The striated extraocular muscles, responsible for eye movements, form the conus. The conus divides the orbit into intraconal and extraconal compartments.

The conus is bounded by seven muscles which insert anteriorly into the orbital sclera and posteriorly into the sheath of the optic nerve:

- four recti muscles: medial (the largest), lateral, superior and inferior
- two oblique muscles: superior and inferior
- levator palpebrae superioris.

Case 1.11

    A Intrahepatic inferior vena cava

    B Gastric lumen

    C Right suprarenal gland

    D Body of L4 vertebra

    E Gluteus medius muscle

Both triangular shaped suprarenal (adrenal) glands can usually be identified lying superior to the upper pole of each kidney. Note the relation of the right suprarenal gland superior and medial to the right kidney. The left suprarenal gland may not be visible at the same axial level as it is often found in a slightly more superior position compared to the right.

Case 1.12

    A Left brachiocephalic vein

    B Right cephalic vein

    C Left internal carotid artery

    D Basilar artery

    E Superior vena cava

This coronal maximum intensity projection (MIP) slab nicely demonstrates the vascular anatomy of the chest and neck.

The cephalic vein joins the axillary vein to form the subclavian vein. The basilar artery is formed by the union of both vertebral arteries.

Case 1.13

    A Right sesamoid bone (in flexor hallucis brevis tendon)

    B Left fourth metatarsophalangeal joint

    C Right navicular bone

    D Tuft of the distal phalanx of the left great toe

    E Left intermediate cuneiform bone

Remember to name the side of the labelled structure when this information is provided on the image in question. The anatomy exam is testing your understanding of radiological anatomy but is also seeing if you can translate this into a report that is understandable by clinicians.

The osseous anatomy of the mid- and forefoot is fundamental knowledge and if you are struggling with this question please refer back to an anatomy text/atlas.

Case 1.14

  A Falx cerebri

  B Interhemispheric fissure

  C Occipital horn of the right lateral ventricle

  D Superior sagittal sinus

  E Cavum septum pellucidum et vergae

Septum pellucidum separates the anterior horns and bodies of the lateral ventricles. It consists of two laminae which attach anteriorly to the corpus callosum and posteriorly to the fornix.

In neonates, there is a narrow cavity between the laminae which does not communicate with the subarachnoid space, called cavum septum pellucidum (CSP). Over 85% of them fuse by 3–6 months of age. In the remaining 15%, the CSP persists as a normal anatomical variant.

Cavum septum pellucidum et vergae is a variant of CSP in which it continues posteriorly, inferior to the splenium and superior fornix.

Case 1.15

  A Mitral valve (anterior leaflet)

  B Muscular portion of interventricular septum

  C Tricuspid valve (anterior leaflet)

  D Left inferior pulmonary vein

  E Spinal cord

Note that the septal leaflet of the mitral valve inserts into the septum at a different level to the septal leaflet of the tricuspid valve, being located more inferiorly towards the right ventricle. This is an important normal anatomical relationship and this offset should be looked for when performing a fetal heart scan at 18 weeks gestation. Tricuspid and mitral leaflets at the same level are often an indication of serious septal defects, e.g. atrioventricular defects. Also note that with this normal offset relationship, there is the potential for a septal defect to occur between the left ventricle and the right atrium, a rare occurrence known as a Gerbode defect.

Case 1.16

  A Right hemidiaphragm

  B Left main bronchus

  C Aortic arch

  D Left clavicle

  E T10

There are three main diaphragmatic hiatuses: the caval hiatus at T8 (most anterior); the oesophageal hiatus at T10 (middle); and the aortic hiatus at T12 (most posterior). The oesophagus is normally indented at several points along its length by anatomical structures. The most inferior of these is at the oesophageal hiatus, caused by a diaphragmatic impression. The left atrium causes a longer impression above this; due to this anatomical relationship, contrast swallow examinations have been used as a means of diagnosing left atrial enlargement. Superiorly to this a combination of the aortic arch and the left main bronchus cause an indentation in the left anterior aspect of the oesophagus.

Case 1.17

A L4/L5 intervertebral disc

B Right pectineus muscle

C Right iliotibial band/tract

D Left obturator internus muscle

E Right gracilis muscle

The iliotibial band is a lateral fibrous tract which originates from the iliac tubercle and inserts into the lateral condyle of the tibia. Due to its fibrous nature, it is distinctively shown as a low signal band on the lateral aspect of the thigh within the subcutaneous fat.

The pectineus muscle originates from the pectineal line of the pubis and inserts into the pectineal line of the superomedial femur – remember pectineus = PPP.

Case 1.18

A Right external auditory canal

B Right carotid canal

C Right zygomatic arch

D Left nasal bone

E Left jugular foramen

The petrous portion of the temporal bone contains two important foramina:

The jugular foramen lies inferior to the middle ear cavity and posterior to the carotid canal. It transmits the jugular vein and glossopharyngeal (CN IX), vagus (CN X) and accessory (CN XI) cranial nerves. Jugular foramina often differ in size, with the right usually larger than the left.

The carotid canal lies anteromedial to the jugular foramen in the petrous apex. It transmits the internal carotid artery from the neck to the cranium.

Case 1.19

  A Tectorial membrane

  B Posterior arch of C1

  C Transverse ligament

  D Posterior longitudinal ligament

  E Ligamentum flavum

A range of ligaments are involved in maintaining the stability of the spine and in particular the craniocervical junction. The posterior longitudinal ligament runs up the posterior aspects of the vertebral bodies and intervertebral discs, being continuous with the tectorial membrane superiorly which blends with dura at the level of foramen magnum. The transverse ligament arches across the C1 ring to support the odontoid peg. Fibres from the midpoint of this ligament pass superiorly and inferiorly to form the cruciate ligament. Ligamentum flavum connects laminae of adjacent vertebrae from the level of C2–S1. Hypertrophy of this ligament may be evident on MRI as a potential cause of neurological symptoms.

Case 1.20

  A Olecranon

  B Medial epicondyle

  C Trochlea

  D Radial head

  E Capitulum

In a patient of this age (9 years old), typically the only ossification centre not yet visible is the lateral epicondyle (usually visible at approximately 11 years of age). The olecranon is usually more readily identifiable on the lateral radiograph but can be clearly seen here. The mnemonic **CRITOL** can be used to help remember the order in which different ossification centres become visible, which can be very important in the context of trauma. The order is usually **C**apitulum (approximately 1 year of age), **R**adial head (3 years of age), **I**nternal (medial) epicondyle (5 years of age), **T**rochlea (7 years of age), **O**lecranon (9 years of age) and **L**ateral epicondyle (11 years of age). The numerical sequence 1 – 3 – 5 – 7 – 9 – 11 is a useful approximation of the age at which each centre begins to ossify.

Chapter 2

Mock paper 2

20 cases to be answered in 75 minutes

Case 2.1

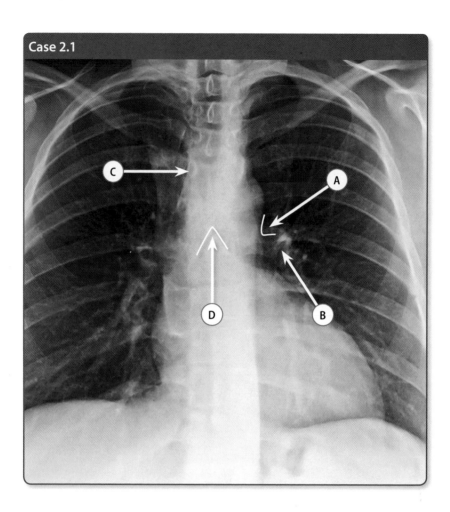

Case 2.1

QUESTION		WRITE YOUR ANSWER HERE
A	Name the structure labelled A.	
B	Name the vascular structure labelled B.	
C	Name the structure labelled C.	
D	Name the outlined structure labelled D.	
E	Which anatomical variant is present on this image?	

To maintain safe flow in the Trust and support ED there is a requirement to discharge sufficient numbers of patients to accommodate those being admitted. This equates to 15-20% of inpatients 7 days per week (~5 patients per 28 bedded ward). Therefore, there is a real need to reconsider our discharge threshold from hospital and use of continuing care and support available in the community. As well as managing your sickest patients, there is also a requirement to identify and prioritise as safely as possible the discharge of patients under your care who are least unwell. There are many options to care for patients outside of the hospital. The Trust is expanding virtual wards, tele-medicine, hot clinics, community assessments and referrals to the Rapid Access to Social Care (RASC) teams. We need to ensure we are optimizing use of these facilities to ensure that access and safe care is maintained.

We wish to re-enforce our assurances of corporate and professional support for clinical decisions made under severe operational pressure. Recognising that staff shortages due to sickness are also likely. We recognise that you are likely to have concerns about both the professional practicalities and implications of working under sustained pressure. We are committed to doing what we can to ensure you are supported and safe.

Chairman: Professor Steve Field CBE
Chief Executive: Professor David Loughton CBE
Preventing Infection - Protecting Patients

A Teaching Trust of the University of Birmingham

Safe & Effective | Kind & Caring | Exceeding Expectation

SMOKEFREE

We are confident all staff will continue to respond and carry out their duties professionally, informed by the values and principles set out in our professional standards. We are sure you will have a clear focus on the individuals you are caring for, but also for those people in the wider system and community who may also need care and treatment.

We all need to support one another during this time, ensuring that as part of a team, we recognize the impact of coping in challenging circumstances, providing support and advice as it's needed. It is, and is going to remain, challenging, and mutual support between professionals is essential. Asking for help from others when you need it is good professional practice. We ask that you also seek support from ourselves if you need it.

Finally, we would like to thank you again for all the extraordinary efforts you have and continue to make in exceptionally difficult circumstances to provide the best possible care for your patients.

Yours sincerely

Prof David Loughton CBE
Group Chief Executive
Officer

Prof Ann-Marie Cannaby
Group Chief Nursing
Officer

Dr Jonathan Odum
Group Chief Medical Officer

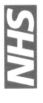

NHS

The Royal Wolverhampton
NHS Trust

New Cross Hospital
Wolverhampton Road
Wolverhampton
West Midlands
WV10 0QP

Tel: 01902 307999

12 January 2023

344 A

Dr Hira Sami
37 Caversham Place
SUTTON COLDFIELD
B73 6HW

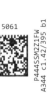

5061

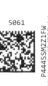

P444SSM221FW
A344 c1.42/395 b1

Dear Hira

You will be aware of the current pressures within the NHS. The stories in the media are very real across the UK and in Wolverhampton.

Quite rightly, the immediate focus is on our urgent / emergency care services and the impact on the ambulance service being able to offload patients into ED in a timely manner. The need for our urgent and emergency care to function effectively is not only to minimise patient harm for non-elective

Case 2.2

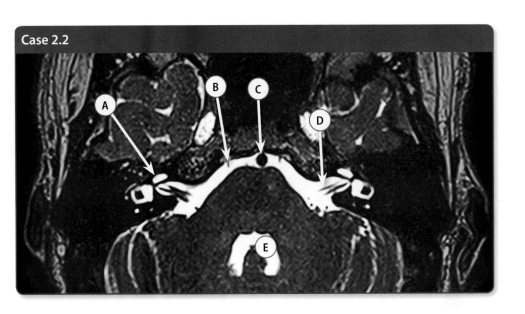

Case 2.2

QUESTION		WRITE YOUR ANSWER HERE
A	Name the structure labelled A.	
B	Name the structure labelled B.	
C	Name the structure labelled C.	
D	Name the structure labelled D.	
E	Name the CSF space labelled E.	

Case 2.3

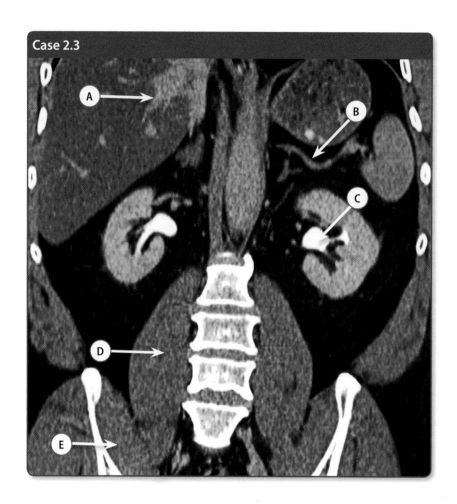

Case 2.3

QUESTION		WRITE YOUR ANSWER HERE
A	Name the structure labelled A.	
B	Name the structure labelled B.	
C	Name the structure labelled C.	
D	Name the structure labelled D.	
E	Name the structure labelled E.	

Case 2.4

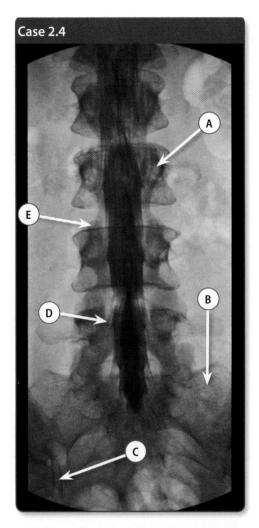

Case 2.4

QUESTION		WRITE YOUR ANSWER HERE
A	Name the structure labelled A.	
B	Name the structure labelled B.	
C	Name the structure labelled C.	
D	Name the structure labelled D.	
E	Name the structure labelled E.	

Case 2.5

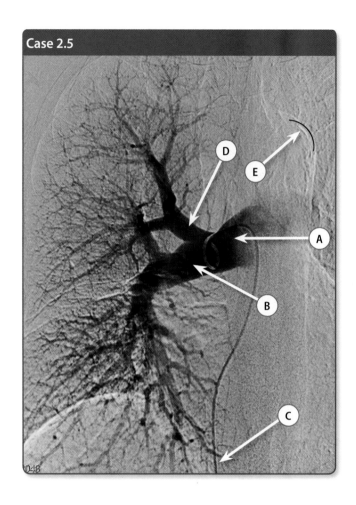

Case 2.5

QUESTION		WRITE YOUR ANSWER HERE
A	Name the structure labelled A.	
B	Name the structure labelled B.	
C	Through which infra-diaphragmatic vessel does the catheter pass through at point C?	
D	Name the structure labelled D.	
E	Name the outlined structure labelled E.	

Case 2.6

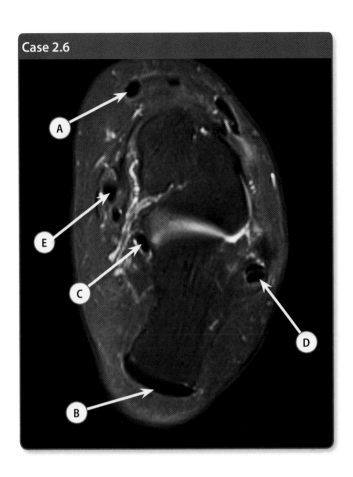

Case 2.6 Axial MRI of the left ankle

QUESTION		WRITE YOUR ANSWER HERE
A	Name the structure labelled A.	
B	Name the structure labelled B.	
C	Name the structure labelled C.	
D	What is the insertion site of the structure labelled D?	
E	Name the structure labelled E.	

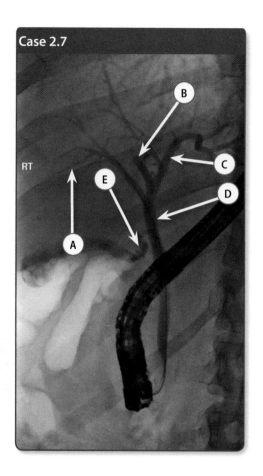

Case 2.7

RT

Case 2.7	
QUESTION	**WRITE YOUR ANSWER HERE**
A Name the structure labelled A.	
B Name the structure labelled B.	
C Name the structure labelled C.	
D Name the structure labelled D.	
E Name the structure labelled E.	

Case 2.8

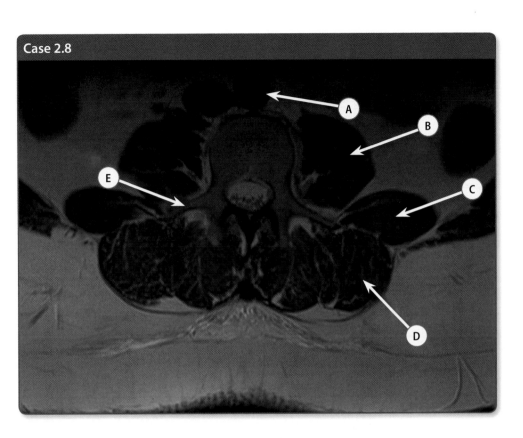

Case 2.8 Axial MRI at the level of L3

QUESTION		WRITE YOUR ANSWER HERE
A	Name the structure labelled A.	
B	Name the structure labelled B.	
C	Name the structure labelled C.	
D	Name the structure labelled D.	
E	Name the structure labelled E.	

Case 2.9

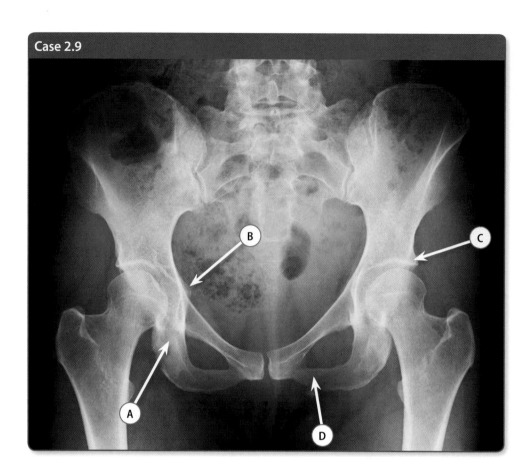

Case 2.9

QUESTION		WRITE YOUR ANSWER HERE
A	Name the structure labelled A.	
B	Name the structure labelled B.	
C	What muscle originates from the structure labelled C?	
D	Name the structure labelled D.	
E	Where is the insertion point of the right iliopsoas muscle?	

Case 2.10

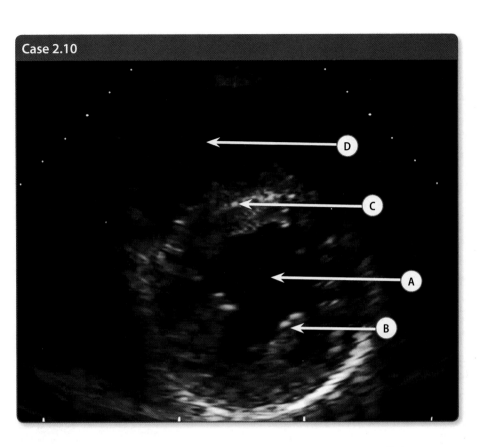

Case 2.10

QUESTION		WRITE YOUR ANSWER HERE
A	Name the chamber labelled A.	
B	Name the structure labelled B.	
C	Name the structure labelled C	
D	Name the chamber labelled D.	
E	How many papillary muscles are usually present in the heart?	

Case 2.11

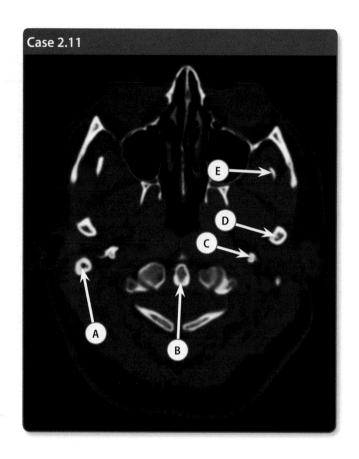

Case 2.11

QUESTION		WRITE YOUR ANSWER HERE
A	Name the structure labelled A.	
B	Name the structure labelled B.	
C	Name the structure labelled C.	
D	Name the structure labelled D.	
E	Name the structure labelled E.	

Case 2.12

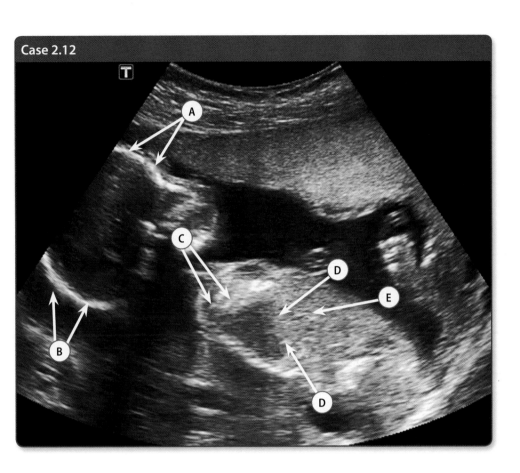

Case 2.12

QUESTION		WRITE YOUR ANSWER HERE
A	Name the structure labelled A.	
B	Name the structure labelled B.	
C	Name the structure labelled C.	
D	Name the structure labelled D.	
E	Name the structure labelled E.	

Case 2.13

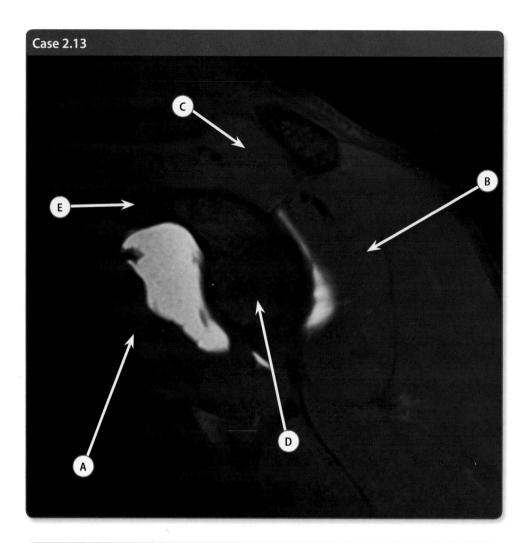

Case 2.13

QUESTION		WRITE YOUR ANSWER HERE
A	Name the structure labelled A.	
B	Name the structure labelled B.	
C	Name the structure labelled C.	
D	Name the structure labelled D.	
E	Name the structure labelled E.	

Case 2.14

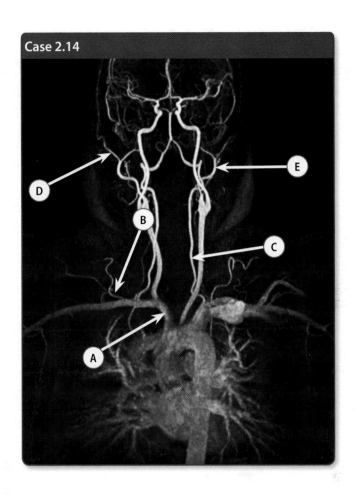

Case 2.14

QUESTION		WRITE YOUR ANSWER HERE
A	Name the structure labelled A.	
B	Name the structure labelled B.	
C	Name the structure labelled C.	
D	Name the structure labelled D.	
E	Name the structure labelled E.	

Case 2.15

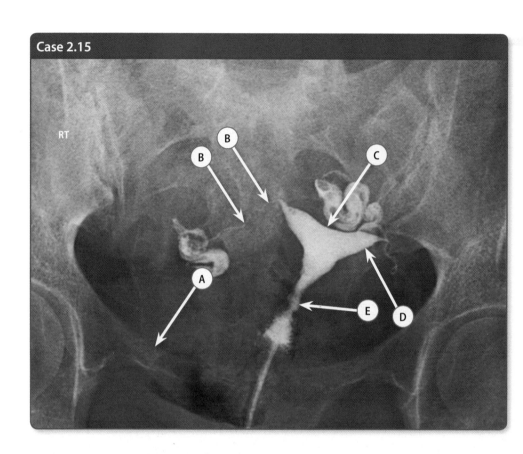

Case 2.15

QUESTION		WRITE YOUR ANSWER HERE
A	Name the structure labelled A.	
B	Name the structure labelled B.	
C	Name the structure labelled C.	
D	Name the structure labelled D.	
E	Name the structure labelled E.	

Case 2.16

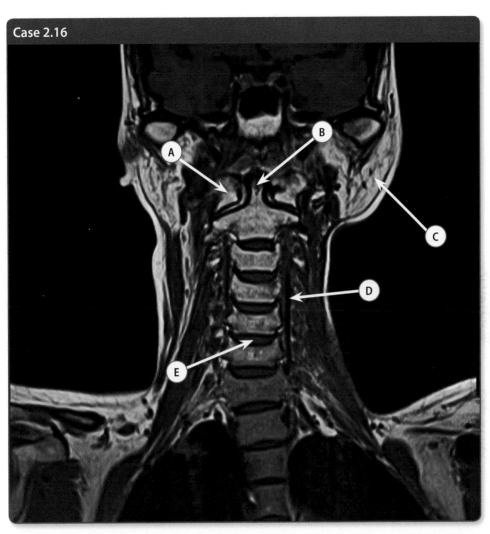

Case 2.16

QUESTION		WRITE YOUR ANSWER HERE
A	Name the structure labelled A.	
B	Name the structure labelled B.	
C	Name the structure labelled C.	
D	Name the structure labelled D.	
E	Name the structure labelled E.	

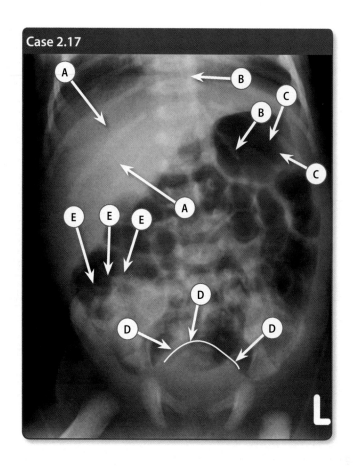

Case 2.17

QUESTION		WRITE YOUR ANSWER HERE
A	Name the structure labelled A.	
B	Name the tube labelled B.	
C	Name the gaseous structure labelled C.	
D	Name the structure outlined by D.	
E	Name the osseous structure labelled E.	

Case 2.18

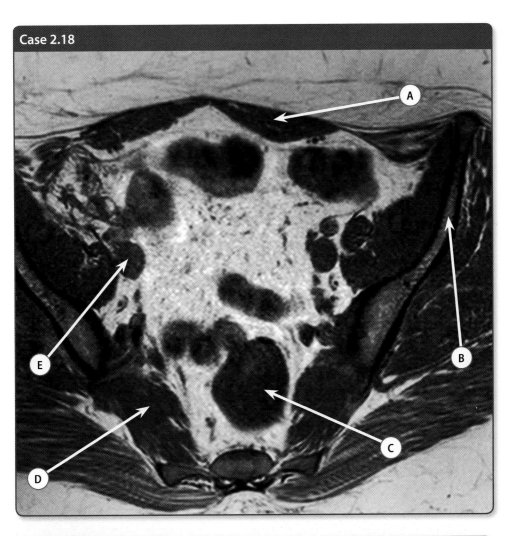

Case 2.18

QUESTION		WRITE YOUR ANSWER HERE
A	Name the structure labelled A.	
B	Name the structure labelled B.	
C	Name the structure labelled C.	
D	Name the structure labelled D.	
E	Name the structure labelled E.	

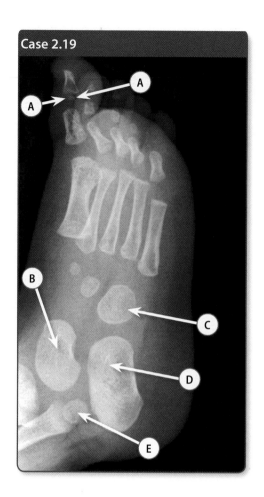

Case 2.19

Case 2.19		
QUESTION		**WRITE YOUR ANSWER HERE**
A	Name the structure labelled A.	
B	Name the structure labelled B.	
C	Name the structure labelled C.	
D	Name the structure labelled D.	
E	Name the structure labelled E.	

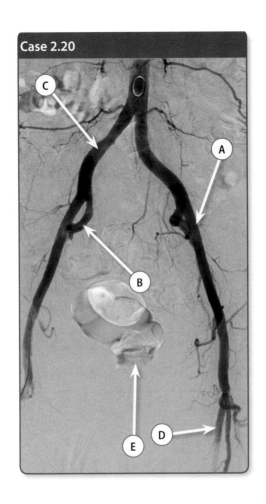

Case 2.20

Case 2.20

QUESTION		WRITE YOUR ANSWER HERE
A	Name the structure labelled A.	
B	Name the structure labelled B.	
C	Name the structure labelled C.	
D	Name the structure labelled D.	
E	Name the structure labelled E.	

Answers

Case 2.1

A Aorto-pulmonary angle or aorto-pulmonary window

B Left lower lobe pulmonary artery

C Right pedicle of T5

D Carina

E Azygos lobe/fissure

The aorto-pulmonary angle is an important anatomical landmark formed by the lateral edge of the aorta and the upper margin of the left pulmonary artery. This angle can be obliterated in cases of mediastinal lymph node enlargement. The ligamentum arteriosum and the left recurrent laryngeal nerve are two important structures located here.

Case 2.2

A Right cochlea

B Right abducens (VI) nerve

C Basilar artery

D Left facial (VII) nerve

E Fourth ventricle

3D SPACE is a heavily T2-weighted sequence which renders high quality images depicting the origin and interim course of the cranial nerves arising from the surface of the brain, brainstem and superior spinal cord. Three cranial nerves (VI, VII and VIII) are depicted in this image.

As illustrated in **Figure 2.1**, the anatomical course of the above nerves is as follows:

- VI nerve, which travels to the Dorello canal in the clivus, is the more anterior and thinner one in relation to the VII and VIII cranial nerves

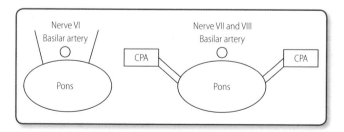

Figure 2.1 Schematic illustration of the cisternal segments of VI, VII and VIII cranial nerves. CPA, cerebellopontine angle.

- VII and VIII nerves, which travel in parallel anterolaterally, course towards the internal auditory meatus, are thicker and situated laterally and posteriorly in relation to the VI nerve
- The basilar artery (BA) and the cerebellopontine angle (CPA) are important anatomic landmarks for orientating yourself.

Case 2.3

A Right hepatic vein

B Splenic artery

C Left renal pelvis

D Right psoas muscle

E Right iliacus muscle

In many institutions, the CT urogram has completely replaced the conventional IVU. The patient is scanned approximately 10–12 minutes after the administration of the intravenous contrast, allowing adequate time for the kidneys to excrete the administered contrast. The excreted contrast can then be seen in the renal collecting systems, ureters and bladder, with tumours being evident as filling defects.

Case 2.4

A Left pedicle of L3

B Left sacral alum

C Right sacro-iliac joint

D Right L5 nerve root

E Right superior articular process of L4

Fluoroscopic lumbar myelography is performed as the initial stage of CT myelography and can also provide useful information as to the presence of intervertebral disc disease and nerve root involvement. Nerve roots are evident as filling defects which exit the spinal cord anterolaterally and course inferolaterally on each side. The conus medullaris can be visualised extending down to the level of L1/2, and the filum terminale may also be identified in the midline. The highest level of the iliac crest (L4) is used as a guide for lumbar puncture, which is usually performed using the interspace of the level above or below.

Case 2.5

A Right pulmonary artery

B Right lower lobe pulmonary artery

C Inferior vena cava

D Right upper lobe pulmonary artery

E Aortic arch

The pulmonary trunk arises from the right ventricular outflow tract. The approach to the pulmonary artery is usually via the femoral vein, the external and common iliac veins and on up the inferior vena cava (IVC) into the right atrium, through the tricuspid valve and right ventricle. The pulmonary valve is crossed before parking the catheter in the pulmonary trunk for angiography.

Hint: an easy way to differentiate between an arterial pulmonary angiogram and a pulmonary venogram is by focusing on the centre of the chest: venography will show contrast in the left atrium whereas pulmonary arteriography will show a lack of contrast in the heart.

Case 2.6

A Left tibialis anterior tendon

B Left Achilles tendon

C Left flexor hallucis longus tendon

D Base of the first metatarsal and medial cuneiform (left)

E Left tibialis posterior tendon

The position and names of the medial flexor tendons of the ankle can be easily remembered using the mnemonic 'Tom, Dick and Harry' which is representative of structures running from medial to lateral:

- **Tom** – posterior **T**ibial tendon
- **Dick** – flexor **D**igitorum longus tendon
- **And** – posterior tibial **A**rtery
- **Harry** – flexor **H**allucis longus tendon

The lateral ankle tendons comprise of the peroneal tendons – longus and brevis. The peroneus brevis tendon lies anterior (sometimes medial) to the peroneus longus tendon.

- Peroneus longus inserts into the base of the first metatarsal and medial cuneiform
- Peroneus brevis inserts into the base of the fifth metatarsal.

Case 2.7

A Right intrahepatic duct

B Right posterior sectoral duct

C Left hepatic duct

D Common hepatic duct

E Cystic duct

This is a single image from an ERCP examination (fluoroscopic imaging of the biliary tract from percutaneous transhepatic cholangiography [PTC] could be shown in the FRCR examination and would look identical, aside from the endoscope). Biliary anatomy is highly variable, with the normal configuration – right anterior and posterior sectoral ducts joining to form right hepatic duct, left hepatic duct joining right hepatic duct to form common hepatic duct, with common bile duct arising when the cystic duct joins the common hepatic duct – present in less than 60% of the population. There is also faint opacification of the gallbladder and filling defects within it, in keeping with gallstones.

Case 2.8

A Abdominal aorta

B Left psoas major muscle

C Left quadratus lumborum muscle

D Left erector spinae muscle

E Right transverse process of L3

The approximate level of lumbar vertebra can be estimated by observing the blood vessels anterior to the vertebral column. The aorta typically bifurcates at the level of L4, with the IVC usually forming at L5 – hence visualisation of both vessels implies a vertebral level of L3 or above. Exam questions commonly enquire as to the exiting nerve root levels. In the lumbar spine, as with thoracic, nerve roots exit under the pedicle of the corresponding vertebra, i.e. the left L3 nerve root exits under the left pedicle of the L3 vertebra, through the neural exit foramen. This is an important concept to understand when assessing nerve root compression in intervertebral disc disease.

Case 2.9

A Right ischial ramus

B Right ischial spine

C Left rectus femoris

D Left inferior pubic ramus

E Right lesser trochanter

Knowledge of the muscular and tendinous attachments in the bony pelvis is important given their clinical relevance (not least in the context of avulsion fractures, particularly in adolescent patients) and this is frequently assessed in examinations.

Iliopsoas is formed from psoas major and iliacus, which merge to pass under the iliac ligament to insert onto the lesser trochanter. Iliopsoas is the most powerful hip flexor and can avulse the lesser trochanter.

Rectus femoris originates from the anterior inferior iliac spine whereas sartorius arises from the anterior superior iliac spine (as does tensor fascia lata).

The hamstring origin is the ischial tuberosity and is the most common avulsion site in the pelvis.

Case 2.10

A Left ventricle

B Papillary muscle

C Interventricular septum

D Right ventricle

E Five

This is a parasternal short axis echocardiographic view of the left ventricle at the level of the papillary muscles which demonstrates the circumferential configuration of the left ventricle. Similar views are also obtained at the level of the mitral valve. The right ventricle is lies anterior to the left ventricle.

There are three papillary muscles in the right ventricle and two in the left ventricle.

Case 2.11

A Right mastoid process

B Odontoid process of axis (C2)

C Left styloid process of the temporal bone

D Left condylar process of the mandible

E Left coronoid process of the mandible

The bony processes of the skull and facial bones serve as anchor points for muscular and ligamentous attachments. The following are visible at the level of the cranio-cervical junction:

- **Mastoid process** – conical projection of the mastoid portion of the temporal bone. It serves as an insertion for sternocleidomastoid, splenius capitis and longissimus capitis muscles.
- **Styloid process** – arises from the inferior surface of the temporal bone. The point of insertion for styloglossus, stylohyoid and stylopharyngeus muscles.
- **Condylar process** – posterior process of the mandible forming the temporomandibular joint. It contains a small tubercle superiorly for the temporomandibular ligament attachment.
- **Coronoid process** – projection from the mandible. The point of insertion for the temporalis muscle.
- **Odontoid process** – superior protuberance of the axis, articulating with the anterior arch of the atlas. Its apex serves as an attachment point for the apical odontoid ligament and the alar ligaments.

Case 2.12

A Frontal bone

B Occipital bone

C Ribs

D Diaphragm

E Liver

In the second trimester, bones of the skull vault are visualised as echogenic lines. Certain calvarial measurements can be taken to assess fetal age, in particular the biparietal diameter. This should be no more than 90% of the occipitofrontal diameter, giving an overall oval shape to the skull. This is best imaged on axial ultrasound, although frontal and occipital bones are clearly visualised here. The ribs are seen as echogenic lines; the clavicles can also be clearly identified at this gestational age but are better identified on axial imaging.

Case 2.13

A Subscapularis muscle

B Infraspinatus muscle

C Supraspinatus muscle

D Glenoid of scapula

E Coracoid process of scapula

The following is key knowledge for the rotator cuff:

1. Supraspinatus muscle

   • Origin – supraspinatus fossa of scapula (dorsal, superior to the spine of scapula)
   • Insertion – superior part of the greater tuberosity of ipsilateral humerus.

2. Infraspinatus muscle

   • Origin – infraspinatus fossa of scapula (dorsal, inferior to the spine of scapula)
   • Insertion – middle part of the greater tuberosity of ipsilateral humerus.

3. Subscapularis muscle

   • Origin – subscapular fossa of scapula (ventral surface of body of scapula)
   • Insertion – lesser tuberosity of ipsilateral humerus.

4. Teres minor muscle

   • Origin – lateral scapular angle
   • Insertion – inferior part of the greater tuberosity of ipsilateral humerus.

Remember, the coracoid process is always directed anteriorly, thus allowing you to differentiate the dorsal and ventral musculature of the rotator cuff.

Case 2.14

A Brachiocephalic (innominate) artery

B Right costocervical trunk

C Left vertebral artery

D Right superficial temporal artery

E Left external carotid artery

The costocervical trunk is a branch of the subclavian artery. This can be seen dividing into the deep cervical artery and the supreme intercostal artery. The superficial temporal artery is a terminal branch of the external carotid artery, the other being the maxillary artery.

On the current image, the right thyrocervical trunk is seen to arise adjacent to the right vertebral artery.

Case 2.15

A Right superior pubic ramus

B Isthmus of right fallopian tube

C Uterine fundus

D Left uterine cornu

E Cervical canal

Hysterosalpingography is performed to assess structural causes of infertility and demonstrates the anatomy of the uterine cavity and fallopian tubes. The fallopian tube isthmus is narrow, with contrast passing through here to the wider ampulla, before spilling into the peritoneal cavity.

Case 2.16

A Right lateral mass of atlas

B Odontoid process (peg) of axis

C Left parotid gland

D Left vertebral artery

E C5/6 intervertebral disc

The craniocervical junction consists of the occipital condyles and the first two cervical vertebrae: the atlas (C1) and axis (C2).

The atlas (C1) is an osseous ring with no true body. Its name is derived from the Greek mythological character Atlas, known for carrying the world on his shoulders. This analogy is similar to the human atlas which essentially carries the head on its lateral masses. The atlas articulates with the occipital condyles at the atlanto-occipital joints and with the axis at the atlanto-axial joints.

The axis (C2) has a superior process called the odontoid peg (dens), which is a remnant of the body of C1. There are three articulations between C1 and C2:

- Paired atlanto-axial joints between the lateral masses of C1 and C2 bilaterally
- Unpaired joint between anterior arch of C1 and odontoid process of C2.

Case 2.17

A Liver

B Nasogastric tube

C Fundus of stomach

D Urinary bladder

E Right iliac crest

On this radiograph, of a one day old infant, the urinary bladder and liver are both made conspicuous as a result of the bowel gas pattern, with gaseous bowel running along the inferior edge of the liver and over the dome of the urinary bladder. This feature is useful for assessing for the presence of organomegaly or abdominopelvic masses, which result in abnormal displacement of bowel loops.

Case 2.18

A Left rectus abdominis muscle

B Left iliac wing

C Rectum

D Right piriformis muscle

E Right common iliac vein

Immediately posterior to the lateral aspect of the rectus abdominis muscles lie a collection of small round structures (three on each side in this case), the inferior epigastric vessels.

The sciatic nerve emerges from the pelvis just inferior to the piriformis muscle, via the greater sciatic notch. It descends vertically about halfway between the ischial tuberosity and the greater trochanter of the femur, deep to the gluteus maximus muscle.

Case 2.19

A Epiphysis of distal phalanx of great toe

B Talus

C Cuboid

D Calcaneum

E Distal fibular epiphysis

This is an oblique radiograph of the foot of an 18-month-old child. As would be expected for a patient of this age, the calcaneum, talus and cuboid are the most well-developed talar bones (having commenced ossification during fetal life). The ossification centre of the lateral cuneiform (the first of the cuneiforms to ossify) is better developed than the intermediate cuneiform. The medial cuneiform normally begins to ossify nearer 3 years of age, hence is not visualised on this radiograph.

Case 2.20

A Left external iliac artery

B Right internal iliac artery

C Right common iliac artery

D Left superficial femoral artery

E Rectum (gas filled)

Here is a very simplistic representation of the pelvic arterial tree:

Aorta → common iliac artery

Common iliac artery → bifurcates into internal and external iliac arteries

External iliac artery → common femoral artery (extension of the external iliac artery beyond the inguinal ligament)

Common femoral artery → bifurcates into profunda femoris and superficial femoral arteries

Chapter 3

Mock paper 3

20 cases to be answered in 75 minutes

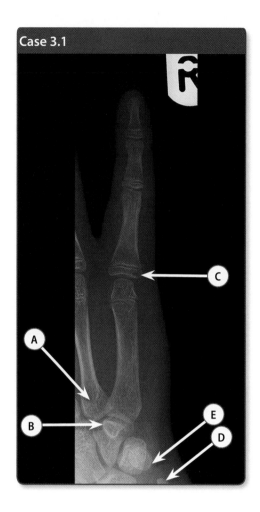

Case 3.1

Case 3.1

	QUESTION	WRITE YOUR ANSWER HERE
A	Name the structure labelled A.	
B	Name the structure labelled B.	
C	Name the structure labelled C.	
D	Name the structure labelled D.	
E	Name the structure labelled E.	

Case 3.2

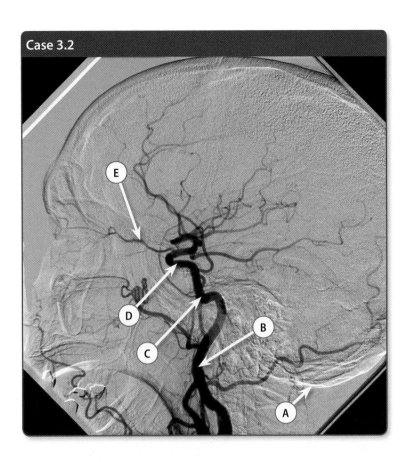

Case 3.2

QUESTION		WRITE YOUR ANSWER HERE
A	Name the osseous structure labelled A.	
B	Name the ICA segment labelled B.	
C	Name the ICA segment labelled C.	
D	Name the ICA segment labelled D.	
E	Name the artery labelled E.	

Case 3.3

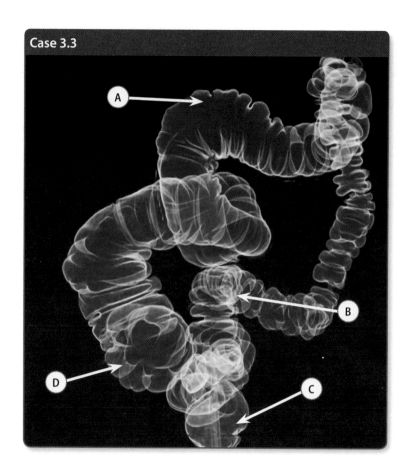

Case 3.3

QUESTION		WRITE YOUR ANSWER HERE
A	Name the structure labelled A.	
B	Name the structure labelled B.	
C	Name the structure labelled C.	
D	Name the structure labelled D.	
E	What is the blood supply of the proximal transverse colon?	

Case 3.4

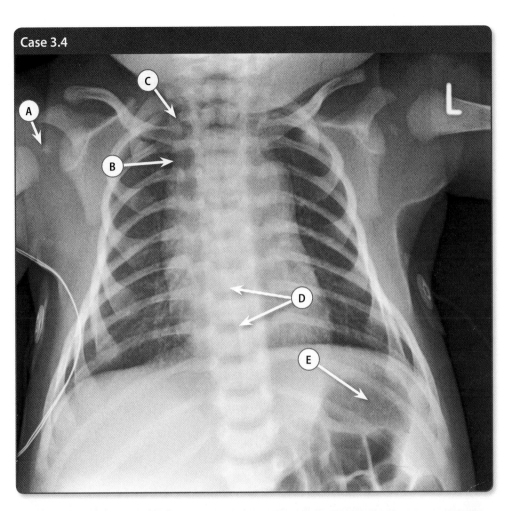

Case 3.4

QUESTION		WRITE YOUR ANSWER HERE
A	Name the structure labelled A.	
B	Name the anterior mediastinal structure labelled B.	
C	Name the structure labelled C.	
D	What does the line labelled D correspond to?	
E	Name the structure labelled E.	

Case 3.5

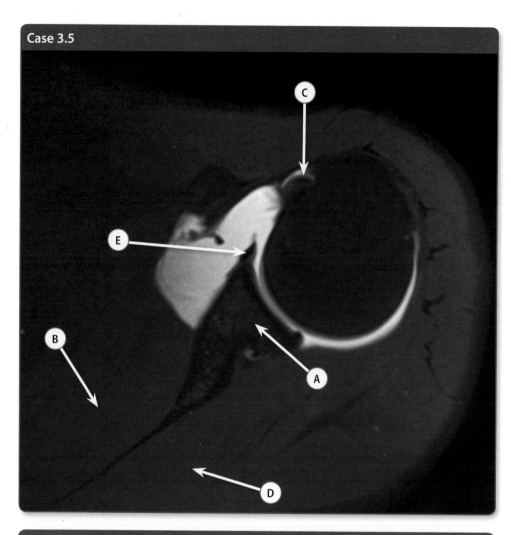

Case 3.5

QUESTION		WRITE YOUR ANSWER HERE
A	Name the structure labelled A.	
B	Name the structure labelled B.	
C	Name the origin of the structure labelled C.	
D	Name the structure labelled D.	
E	Name the structure labelled E.	

Case 3.6

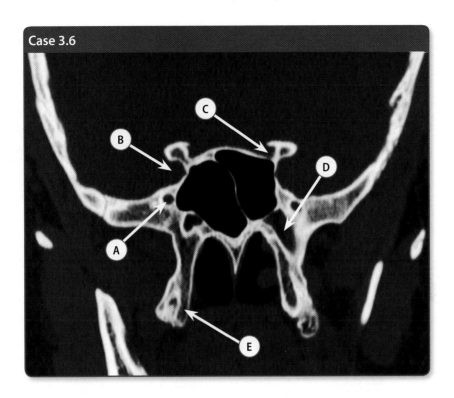

Case 3.6

QUESTION		WRITE YOUR ANSWER HERE
A	Name the structure labelled A.	
B	Name the fissure labelled B.	
C	Name the structure labelled C.	
D	Name the structure labelled D.	
E	Name the structure labelled E.	

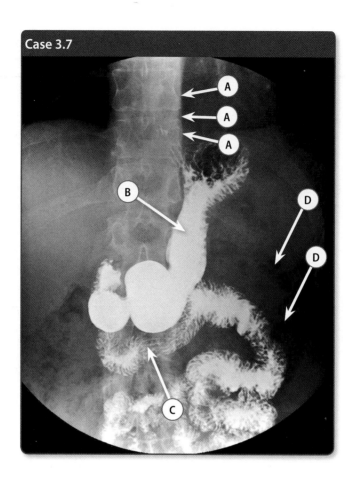

Case 3.7

Case 3.7		
QUESTION		**WRITE YOUR ANSWER HERE**
A	What name is given to line A?	
B	Which unpaired artery arising from the aorta supplies structure B?	
C	Which unpaired artery arising from the aorta supplies structure C?	
D	In what part of the bowel does the gas labelled D lie?	
E	Which part of the duodenum is intraperitoneal?	

Case 3.8

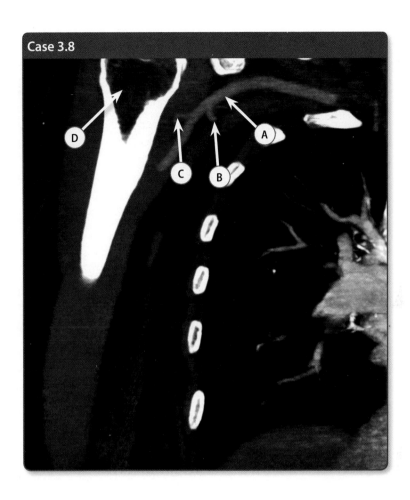

Case 3.8

QUESTION		WRITE YOUR ANSWER HERE
A	Name the structure labelled A.	
B	Name the structure labelled B.	
C	Name the structure labelled C.	
D	Name the structure labelled D.	
E	How many named branches does the axillary artery usually have?	

Case 3.9

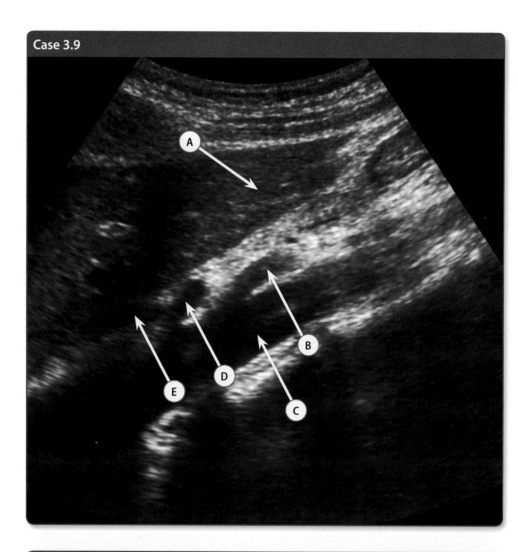

Case 3.9

QUESTION		WRITE YOUR ANSWER HERE
A	Name the structure labelled A.	
B	Name the structure labelled B.	
C	Name the structure labelled C.	
D	Name the structure labelled D.	
E	Name the structure labelled E.	

Case 3.10

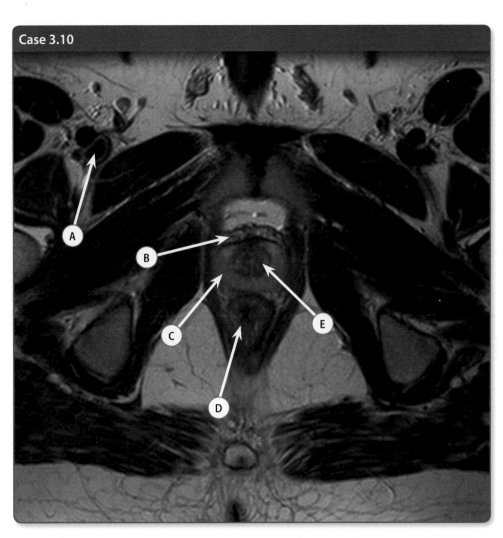

Case 3.10

QUESTION		WRITE YOUR ANSWER HERE
A	Name the structure labelled A.	
B	Name the structure labelled B.	
C	Name the structure labelled C.	
D	Name the structure labelled D.	
E	Name the structure labelled E.	

Case 3.11

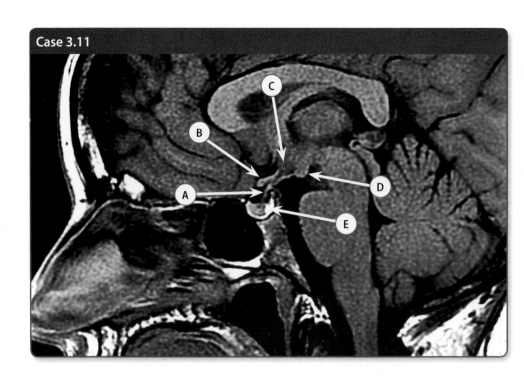

Case 3.11

QUESTION		WRITE YOUR ANSWER HERE
A	Name the structure labelled A.	
B	Name the structure labelled B.	
C	Name the structure labelled C.	
D	Name the structure labelled D.	
E	Name the structure labelled E.	

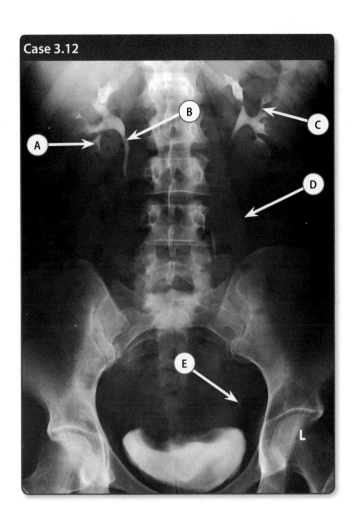

Case 3.12

	Case 3.12	
QUESTION		**WRITE YOUR ANSWER HERE**
A	Name the structure labelled A.	
B	Name the structure labelled B.	
C	Name the structure labelled C.	
D	What does the line labelled D correspond to?	
E	Name the structure labelled E.	

Case 3.13

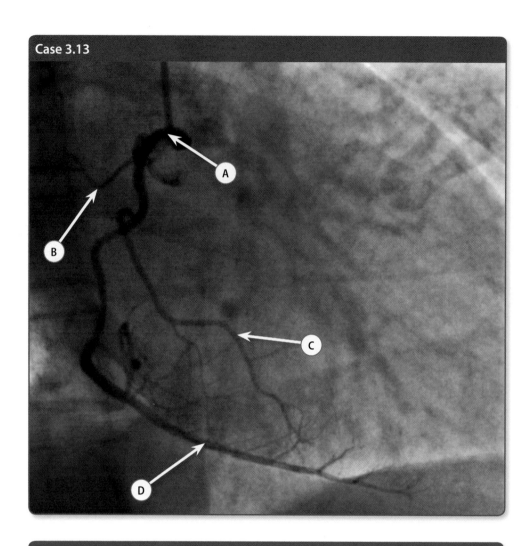

Case 3.13

QUESTION		WRITE YOUR ANSWER HERE
A	Name the structure labelled A.	
B	Name the structure labelled B.	
C	Name the structure labelled C.	
D	Name the structure labelled D.	
E	What determines coronary artery dominance?	

Case 3.14

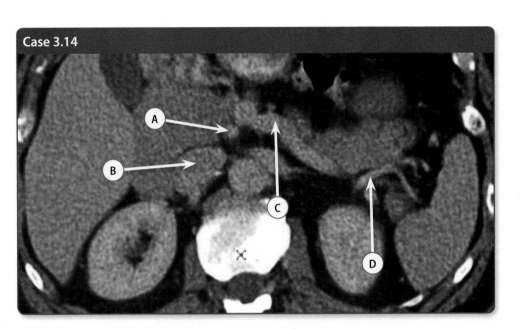

Case 3.14

QUESTION		WRITE YOUR ANSWER HERE
A	Name the structure labelled A.	
B	Name the structure labelled B.	
C	Name the structure labelled C.	
D	Name the structure labelled D.	
E	Which anatomical variant is present on this image?	

Case 3.15

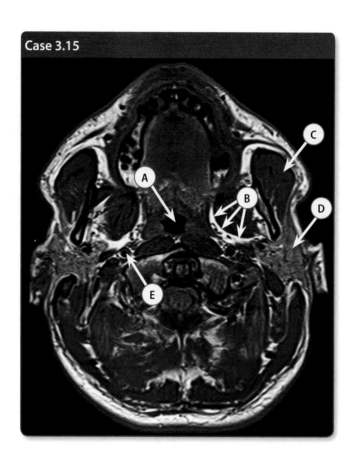

Case 3.15

QUESTION		WRITE YOUR ANSWER HERE
A	Name the structure labelled A.	
B	Name the space labelled B.	
C	Name the structure labelled C.	
D	Name the structure labelled D.	
E	Name the structure labelled E.	

Case 3.16

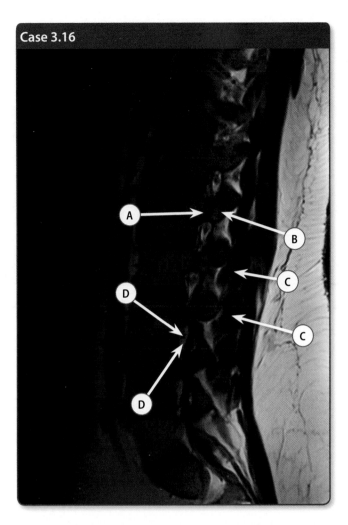

Case 3.16

QUESTION		WRITE YOUR ANSWER HERE
A	Name the structure labelled A.	
B	Name the structure labelled B.	
C	Name the structure labelled C.	
D	Name the structure labelled D.	
E	What nerve root exits below the left L4 pedicle?	

Case 3.17

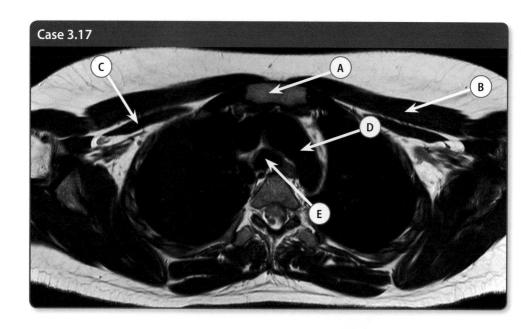

Case 3.17

QUESTION		WRITE YOUR ANSWER HERE
A	Name the structure labelled A.	
B	Name the structure labelled B.	
C	Name the structure labelled C.	
D	Name the structure labelled D.	
E	Name the structure labelled E.	

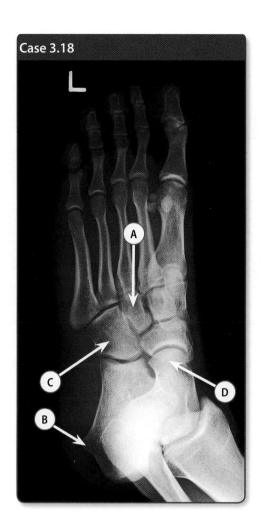

Case 3.18

Case 3.18

QUESTION		WRITE YOUR ANSWER HERE
A	Name the structure labelled A.	
B	Name the structure labelled B.	
C	Name the structure labelled C.	
D	Name the structure labelled D.	
E	Which anatomical variant is present on this image?	

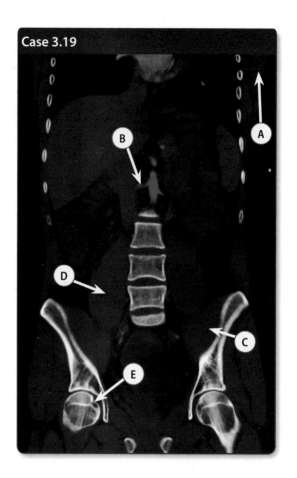

Case 3.19

Case 3.19		
QUESTION		**WRITE YOUR ANSWER HERE**
A	Name the structure labelled A.	
B	Name the structure labelled B.	
C	Name the structure labelled C.	
D	Name the structure labelled D.	
E	What structure inserts at E (fovea)?	

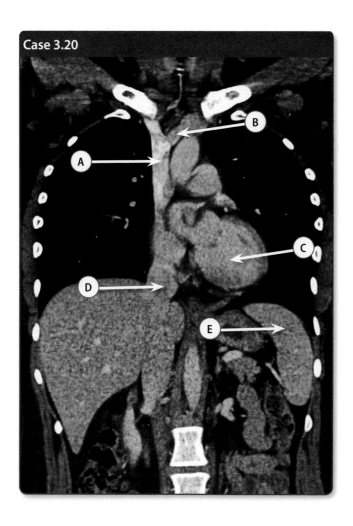

Case 3.20

QUESTION		WRITE YOUR ANSWER HERE
A	Name the structure labelled A.	
B	Name the structure labelled B.	
C	Name the chamber labelled C.	
D	Name the structure labelled D.	
E	Name the structure labelled E.	

Answers

Case 3.1

A Base of the right fourth metacarpal (ring finger)

B Hook of right hamate

C Ossification centre of the proximal phalanx of right little finger

D Styloid process of right ulna

E Right pisiform

Carpal bone anatomy is essential core knowledge. Although the full bony carpus is not demonstrated on this radiograph, you should be able to orientate yourself by:

- the hamate and pisiform being on the ulnar aspect of the wrist
- the fifth digit having three phalanges
- the first digit (thumb) having only two phalanges.

Case 3.2

A Occipital bone

B Cervical portion of internal carotid artery

C Petrous portion of internal carotid artery

D Cavernous portion of internal carotid artery

E Ophthalmic artery

There are two internal carotid artery (ICA) classification systems: anatomical and clinical. The anatomical system subdivides the ICA into four portions which can be appreciated on DSA angiography. The clinical system divides the ICA into seven segments, which can be identified on CT and MR angiography.

The following mnemonic will aid you in memorising the four ICA portions: 'Carotid Parts Cannot be Ignored':

- **C**ervical
- **P**etrous
- **C**avernous
- **I**ntracranial (supraclinoid).

Case 3.3

A Transverse colon

B Sigmoid colon

C Rectum

D Caecum

E Middle colic artery

The colon is divided into the caecum, ascending colon, transverse colon, descending colon, sigmoid colon and rectum. The caecum is the blind-ended area of the colon inferior to the ileocaecal valve. The superior mesenteric artery (SMA) and its branches (ileocolic, right and middle colic arteries) supply up to the distal third of the transverse colon.

Branches of the inferior mesenteric artery (IMA) supply the rest of transverse and descending/sigmoid colon.

The major branches of the IMA can be recalled remembering inferior means **LESS**:

- **L**eft colic
- **S**igmoid branches
- **S**uperior rectal

Case 3.4

A Ossification centre of right humeral head

B Thymus

C Right transverse process of T2

D Azygo-oesophageal recess

E Gastric fundus

A number of anatomical lines, stripes and other interfaces are evident on chest radiographs, deviation of which can be a subtle sign of pathology. The azygo-oesophageal recess is visualised as a result of the different densities of the mediastinum and the posteromedial aspect of the right lower lobe. The recess lies anterior to the vertebral column and posterior or lateral to the oesophagus. Its superior extent is the anterior turn of the azygos vein, with the inferior extent being the aortic hiatus. Pathologies which alter the normal contour of the recess include hiatus hernias, oesophageal tumours and lymph node enlargement.

Case 3.5

A Glenoid of scapula

B Subscapularis muscle

C Superior glenoid tubercle

D Infraspinatus muscle

E Anterior glenoid labrum

The rotator cuff is composed of four muscles and their respective tendons. Its function is to stabilise the glenohumeral joint during dynamic activity.

The following muscles make up the rotator cuff:

1. Supraspinatus:

   - Origin – supraspinatus fossa of scapula (dorsal, superior to the spine of scapula)
   - Insertion – superior part of the greater tuberosity of ipsilateral humerus

2. Infraspinatus:

   - Origin – infraspinatus fossa of scapula (dorsal, inferior to the spine of scapula)
   - Insertion – middle part of the greater tuberosity of ipsilateral humerus

3. Subscapularis:

   - Origin – subscapular fossa of scapula (ventral surface of body of scapula)
   - Insertion – lesser tuberosity of ipsilateral humerus

4. Teres minor:

   - Origin – lateral scapular angle
   - Insertion – inferior part of the greater tuberosity of ipsilateral humerus

The long head of biceps brachii muscle originates from the supraglenoid tubercle.

Case 3.6

A Right foramen rotundum

B Right superior orbital fissure

C Left optic canal

D Left pterygopalatine fossa

E Right medial pterygoid plate

With a bit of imagination, the sphenoid bone on coronal CT resembles a circus bear, with its hind legs pointing upwards (**Figure 3.1**):

- **Ears** – anterior clinoid processes

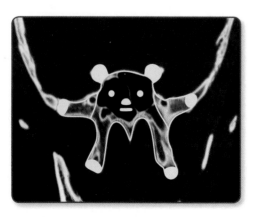

Figure 3.1 The sphenoid bone at the level of the sphenoid sinus.

- **Hind legs** – greater wings of the sphenoid bone
- **Front legs** – medial and lateral pterygoid plates
- **Muzzle** – sphenoid sinus

Case 3.7

   A Left paraspinal line

   B Coeliac axis (with its gastric branches)

   C Superior mesenteric artery

   D Descending colon

   E First part

The left paraspinal line is an important review area on chest radiographs in particular, reflecting the interface between the left lung and pleura with the fat in the posterior mediastinum, left paraspinal muscles and the adjacent soft tissues. Lateral displacement of this line suggests posterior mediastinal pathologies.

The gastrointestinal tract is divided embryologically into foregut (from mouth to the midpoint of the second part of the duodenum), midgut (from termination of foregut up to two-thirds of the way along the transverse colon) and hindgut (from termination of midgut up to and including the upper anal canal). The blood supply reflects the embryology, with foregut being supplied by coeliac axis, midgut by superior mesenteric artery and hindgut by inferior mesenteric artery.

The duodenum is almost entirely retroperitoneal, with only the first part being intraperitoneal. As such, perforation of structure (C) (part 3 of the duodenum) leads to a retroperitoneal air leak which appears radiographically distinct to pneumoperitoneum.

Case 3.8

   A Right axillary artery

   B Right lateral thoracic artery

   C Right anterior circumflex artery

   D Neck of right humerus

   E Six

The subclavian artery continues as the axillary artery at the outer margin of the first rib. The artery is divided into three segments by the pectoralis minor muscle. A useful mnemonic for remembering the branches of the axillary artery is **S**cam **T**he **L**awyers, **S**ave **A** **P**atient. One arterial branch arises from its first part, two from the second and three from the third part.

The six branches of the axillary artery are as follows:

1. Superior thoracic artery

2.   Thoracoacromial artery

3.   Lateral thoracic artery

4.   Subscapular artery

5.   Anterior circumflex artery

6.   Posterior circumflex artery

Case 3.9

A Left lobe of liver

B Superior mesenteric artery

C Aorta

D Coeliac axis

E Portal vein

The relation of the portal vein to the aorta and coeliac axis is well seen on this image. The portal vein is located anteriorly and to the right of the aorta. The portal venous confluence is located just inferior and to the right of the coeliac axis. This should become a very familiar view and you should expect to be able to recognise these major structures on MRI, CT, US and angiography.

Case 3.10

A Right femoral vein

B Retropubic venous plexus

C Peripheral zone of prostate

D Rectum

E Central zone of prostate

This is an axial T2-weighted MRI through the male pelvis. The peripheral zone of the prostate has brighter signal in this sequence and the central zone is darker. Three distinct zones are described (**Table 3.1**) along with fibromuscular stroma. Structure

Table 3.1 Zonal anatomy of the prostate		
Zone	**Location**	**Pathology**
Peripheral	Subcapsular, posterior aspect	• 70% of malignancies arise here
Central	Surrounds ejaculatory ducts	• Around of 3% malignancies arise here
Transition	Surrounds proximal urethra	• Continues to grow throughout life • Is the area in which benign prostatic hyperplasia occurs • Accounts for 20–30% malignancies

(B) is the retropubic venous plexus (of Santorini), an important structure for the urologist performing a prostatectomy.

Case 3.11

A Pituitary infundibulum (stalk)

B Optic chiasm

C Hypothalamus

D Mamillary body

E Posterior lobe of the pituitary gland

The pituitary gland consists of two functionally and anatomically separate lobes: anterior and posterior. The lobes can be distinguished on a T1-weighted image, on which the posterior lobe returns characteristically bright signal due to the presence of neurosecretory granules.

The posterior pituitary lobe is connected to the hypothalamus by the infundibulum (stalk), which transports hormones from both the anterior and the posterior parts of the pituitary gland.

The mamillary bodies form the posterior part of the hypothalamus and separate it from the midbrain.

Case 3.12

A Right lower pole calyx

B Right pelviureteric junction

C Left infundibulum

D Left psoas major outline

E Distal left ureter

Although intravenous urography (IVU) is becoming a less popular imaging modality with the advent of CT urography, the IVU remains a classic examination film and is good for demonstrating anatomy of the urinary tract. The psoas major outlines should be scrutinised in any abdominal radiograph, as loss of this fat plane can be a subtle sign of a bleed into the retroperitoneum, for example.

Case 3.13

A Right coronary artery

B Sinoatrial nodal artery

C Ventricular branches

D Posterior descending artery

E The vessel from which the posterior descending artery originates

The right coronary artery arises from the anterior sinus of Valsalva. In 50–60%, the first branch of the right coronary artery (RCA) is the small conus branch that supplies the right ventricular outflow tract. In 60% a sinoatrial nodal artery arises as the second branch of the RCA, which runs posteriorly to the sinoatrial node. The next branches are called diagonals and they run anteriorly to supply the anterior wall of the right ventricle.

Case 3.14

A Superior mesenteric artery

B Inferior vena cava

C Splenic vein

D Splenic artery

E Partial midgut malrotation

At the level of L1/L2 the splenic vein is seen travelling towards its confluence with the superior mesenteric vein to form the portal vein. At that level, the superior mesenteric artery is expected to lie to the left of the portal confluence. However, here it is seen to be to the right and slightly posterior. This is a case of a partial midgut malrotation. The incidence of this variation is thought to be around 1/500 births and patients may be asymptomatic or present with midgut volvulus, which this variation predisposes to.

Case 3.15

A Oropharynx

B Left parapharyngeal space

C Left masseter muscle

D Left parotid gland

E Right carotid artery

The neck is anatomically divided into spaces, orientated craniocaudally, separated by fascial planes. The spaces are named after anatomical structures they contain or neighbouring landmarks. Once the anatomical spaces become familiar (**Figure 3.2** and **Table 3.2**), the complex anatomy becomes easier to evaluate.

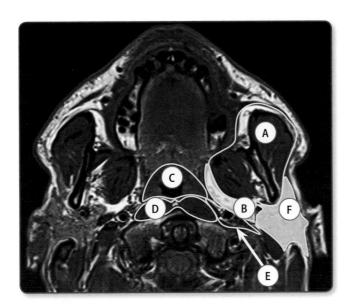

Figure 3.2 T1-weighted axial MRI illustrating anatomical spaces of the neck.

Table 3.2 Content of the anatomical spaces of the neck		
Fig. 3.2 label	**Anatomical space**	**Content**
A	Masticator	Mandible, muscles, trigeminal nerve
B	Parapharyngeal	Fat, maxillary artery, nerves
C	Pharyngeal mucosal	Mucosa, lymphoid tissue, constrictor muscles
D	Retropharyngeal	Fat, pre-cervical muscles
E	Carotid	Carotid artery, jugular vein, lymph nodes, cranial nodes
F	Parotid	Parotid gland, facial nerve, lymph nodes, vessels

Case 3.16

A Left pedicle of L1

B Left pars interarticularis of L1

C Left erector spinae muscle

D L3 neural exit foramen

E Left L4 nerve root

In the cervical spine, nerve roots exit above their correspondingly numbered pedicles. The C8 nerve root has no corresponding vertebra and accordingly exits below the C7 pedicle. In the thoracolumbar spine, nerve roots exit below their correspondingly numbered pedicles. Accordingly, the left L4 nerve root will exit below the left pedicle of L4, in the neural exit foramen formed between the L4 and L5 vertebrae. See the schematic representation of a parasagittal view of the neural exit foramen in **Figure 3.3**.

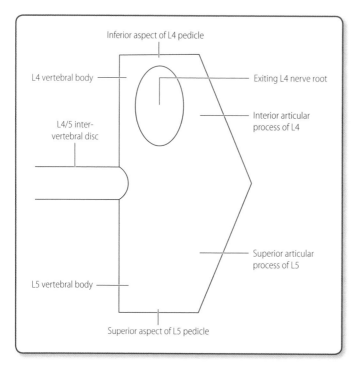

Figure 3.3 Schematic illustration of neural exit foramen.

Case 3.17

   A Sternum

   B Left pectoralis major muscle

   C Right pectoralis minor muscle

   D Aortic arch

   E Trachea

Although the vessel lumina demonstrate flow voids, it should be possible to identify them based on location and relative anatomy. Occasionally, artefacts or pathologies lead to high signal within the blood vessels.

Remember, the airways will also return no signal as they are filled with air.

Case 3.18

  A Left lateral cuneiform

  B Left calcaneal tuberosity

  C Left cuboid

  D Head of left talus

  E Bipartite hallucal sesamoid bone

The hallucal sesamoid bones are present in the majority of the adult population. The most common variant is a bipartite hallucal sesamoid, as shown in this example. It is important to recognise this entity as a variant of normal and for it not to be mistaken as a sesamoid fracture. Bipartite sesamoids will demonstrate smooth, well-corticated margins, whereas fractures will have sharp irregular margins, often with overlying soft tissue swelling.

Case 3.19

  A Left latissimus dorsi muscle

  B Right renal artery

  C Left iliacus muscle

  D Right psoas major muscle

  E Right ligamentum teres

The iliacus muscle arises from the iliac fossa within the pelvis and converges with the psoas major muscle to insert as a unified tendon into the lesser trochanter of the femur. The latissimus dorsi muscle is the broadest muscle of the back and lies on the dorsolateral aspect of the trunk.

The fovea of the femoral head is an indentation which provides the insertion site for ligamentum teres – a stabilising ligament in childhood but a transmitter of arterial supply throughout life.

Case 3.20

  A Superior vena cava

  B Left brachiocephalic vein

  C Left ventricle

  D Suprahepatic inferior vena cava

  E Spleen

This example shows the systemic venous drainage via the large central veins draining into the heart. The superior vena cava (SVC) is almost always right-sided but can occasionally be left-sided or even bilateral.

In the 5th week of intrauterine life, three pairs of major veins can be distinguished: (a) the vitelline, carrying blood from the yolk sac to the sinus venosus; (b) the umbilical veins, carrying oxygenated blood to the embryo; and (c) the cardinal veins, draining the body of the embryo. This system consists of the anterior cardinal veins, which drain the cephalic part of the embryo, and the posterior cardinal veins, which drain the remainder of the embryo. The anterior and posterior veins join before entering the sinus horn and form the common cardinal veins. Formation of the vena cava system is characterised by the appearance of anastomoses between the left and right sides in such a manner that the blood from the left side is channelled to the right side. The anastomosis between the anterior cardinal veins develops into the left brachiocephalic vein. The superior vena cava is formed by the right common cardinal vein and the proximal portion of the right anterior cardinal vein.

Chapter 4

Mock paper 4

20 cases to be answered in 75 minutes

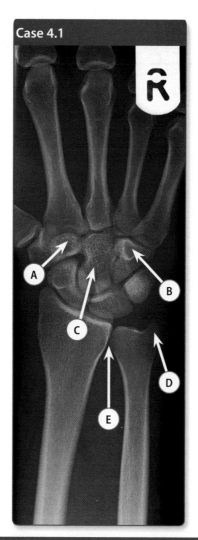

Case 4.1

Case 4.1

QUESTION		WRITE YOUR ANSWER HERE
A	Name the structure labelled A.	
B	Name the structure labelled B.	
C	Name the structure labelled C.	
D	Name the structure labelled D.	
E	Name the structure labelled E.	

Case 4.2

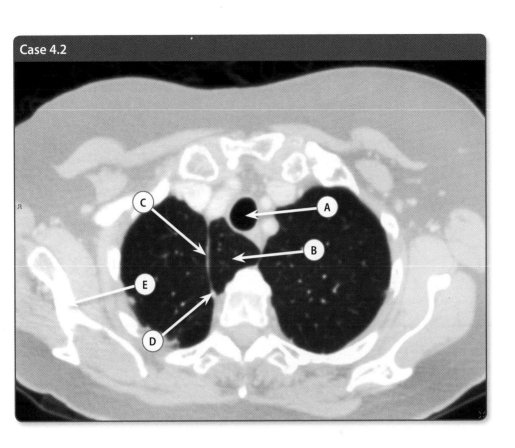

Case 4.2

QUESTION		WRITE YOUR ANSWER HERE
A	Name the structure labelled A.	
B	Name the structure labelled B.	
C	Name the structure labelled C.	
D	Name the structure labelled D.	
E	Name the structure labelled E.	

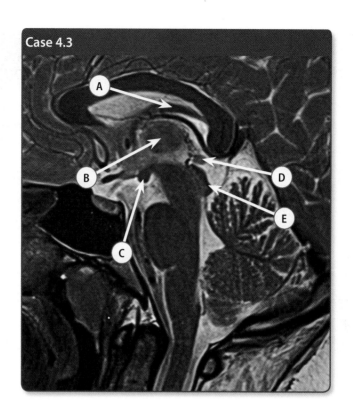

Case 4.3

Case 4.3	
QUESTION	**WRITE YOUR ANSWER HERE**
A Name the structure labelled A.	
B Name the structure labelled B.	
C Name the structure labelled C.	
D Name the structure labelled D.	
E Name the structure labelled E.	

Case 4.4

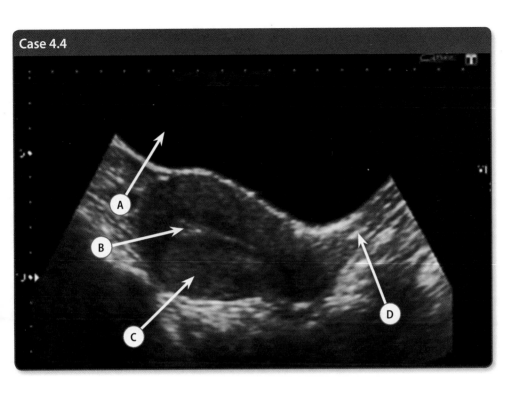

Case 4.4

QUESTION		WRITE YOUR ANSWER HERE
A	Name the structure labelled A.	
B	Name the structure labelled B.	
C	Name the structure labelled C	
D	Name the structure labelled D.	
E	What is the upper limit of normal thickness of the endometrium in a pre-menopausal woman?	

Case 4.5

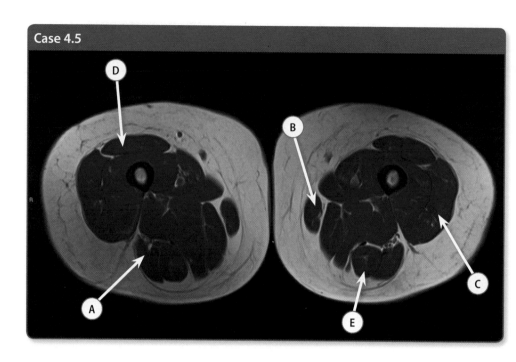

Case 4.5

QUESTION		WRITE YOUR ANSWER HERE
A	Name the structure labelled A.	
B	Name the structure labelled B.	
C	Name the structure labelled C.	
D	Name the structure labelled D.	
E	Name the structure labelled E.	

Case 4.6

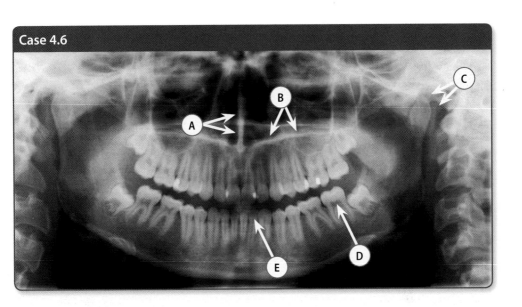

Case 4.6

QUESTION		WRITE YOUR ANSWER HERE
A	Name the structure labelled A.	
B	Name the structure labelled B.	
C	Name the joint labelled C.	
D	Name the structure labelled D.	
E	Name the structure labelled E.	

Case 4.7

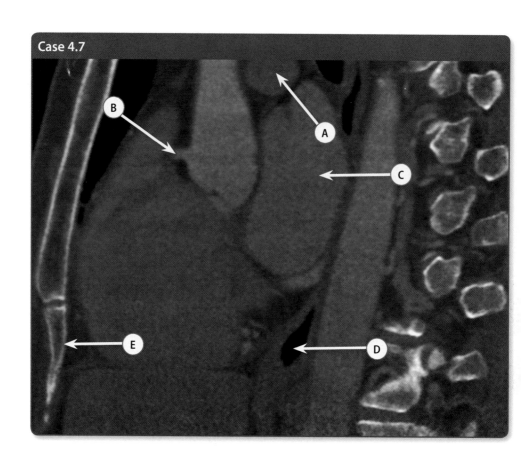

Case 4.7

QUESTION		WRITE YOUR ANSWER HERE
A	Name the structure labelled A.	
B	Name the structure labelled B.	
C	Name the chamber labelled C.	
D	In what structure does the gas labelled D lie?	
E	Name the structure labelled E.	

Case 4.8

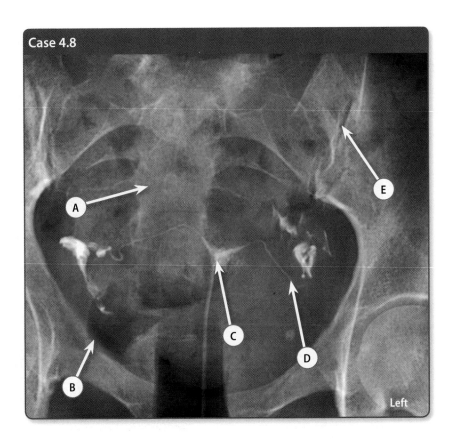

Left

Case 4.8

QUESTION		WRITE YOUR ANSWER HERE
A	Name the structure labelled A.	
B	Name the osseous line labelled B.	
C	Name the structure labelled C.	
D	Name the structure labelled D.	
E	Name the structure labelled E.	

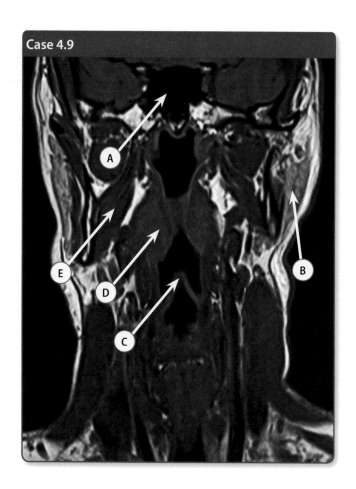

Case 4.9

Case 4.9	
QUESTION	**WRITE YOUR ANSWER HERE**
A Name the structure labelled A.	
B Name the structure labelled B.	
C Name the structure labelled C.	
D Name the structure labelled D.	
E Name the structure labelled E.	

Case 4.10

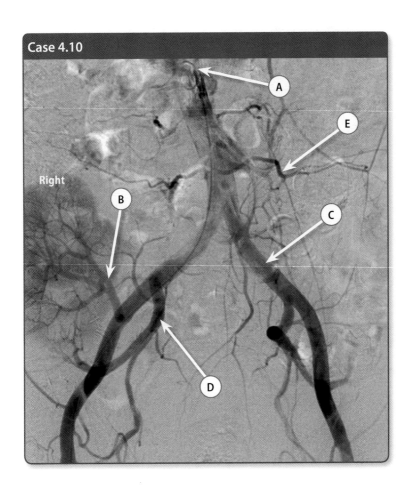

Right

A

E

B

C

D

Case 4.10

QUESTION		WRITE YOUR ANSWER HERE
A	Name the device labelled A.	
B	What organ is the artery labelled B supplying?	
C	Name the structure labelled C.	
D	Name the structure labelled D.	
E	Name the structure labelled E.	

Case 4.11

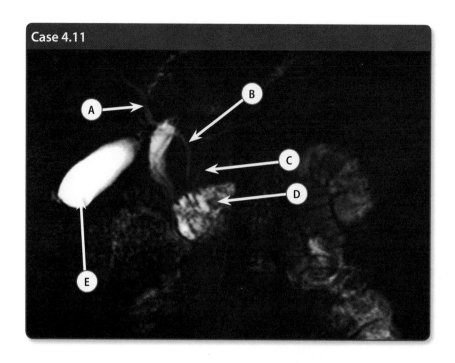

Case 4.11

QUESTION		WRITE YOUR ANSWER HERE
A	Name the structure labelled A.	
B	Name the structure labelled B.	
C	Name the structure labelled C.	
D	Name the structure labelled D.	
E	Name the structure labelled E.	

Case 4.12

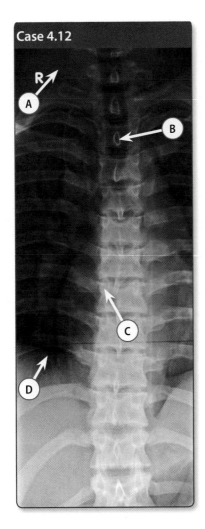

Case 4.12	
QUESTION	**WRITE YOUR ANSWER HERE**
A Name the structure labelled A.	
B Name the structure labelled B.	
C Name the structure labelled C.	
D Name the structure labelled D.	
E Which anatomical variant is present on this image?	

Case 4.13

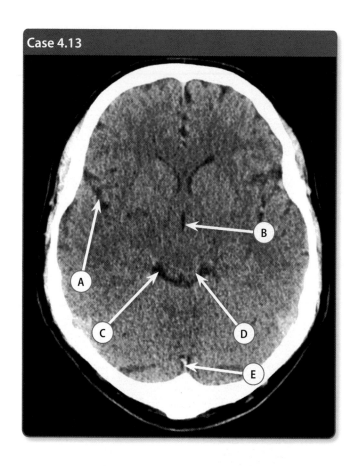

Case 4.13

QUESTION		WRITE YOUR ANSWER HERE
A	Name the structure labelled A.	
B	Name the structure labelled B.	
C	Name the structure labelled C.	
D	Name the structure labelled D.	
E	Name the structure labelled E.	

Case 4.14

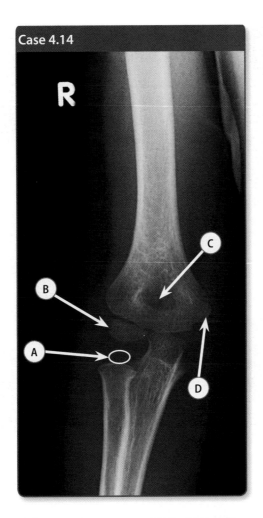

Case 4.14	
QUESTION	**WRITE YOUR ANSWER HERE**
A	Name the structure labelled A.	
B	Name the structure labelled B.	
C	Name the structure labelled C.	
D	Name the structure labelled D.	
E	Which ossification centre is normally the next to develop?	

Case 4.15

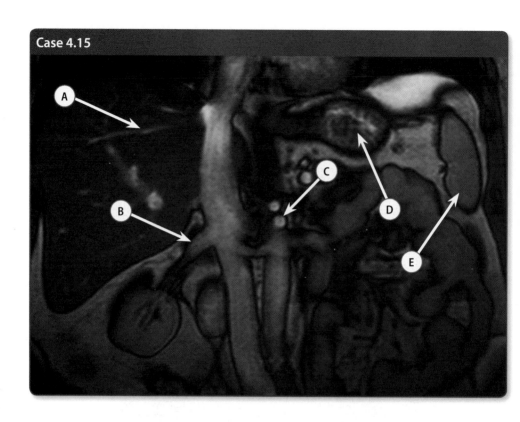

Case 4.15

QUESTION	WRITE YOUR ANSWER HERE
A Name the structure labelled A.	
B Name the structure labelled B.	
C Name the structure labelled C.	
D Name the structure labelled D.	
E Name the structure labelled E.	

Case 4.16

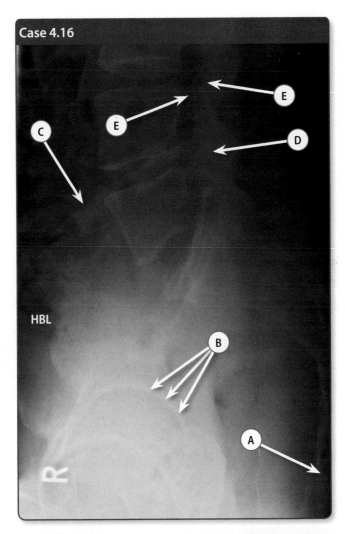

HBL

R

Case 4.16

QUESTION		WRITE YOUR ANSWER HERE
A	Name the structure labelled A.	
B	Name the structure labelled B.	
C	Name the structure labelled C.	
D	Name the structure labelled D.	
E	Name the articulation labelled E.	

Case 4.17

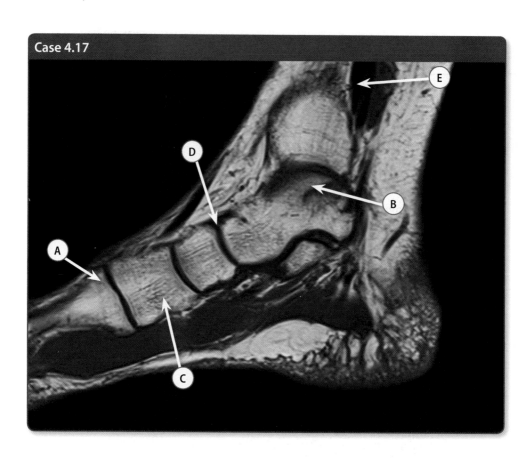

Case 4.17

QUESTION		WRITE YOUR ANSWER HERE
A	Name the structure labelled A.	
B	Name the structure labelled B.	
C	Name the structure labelled C.	
D	Name the structure labelled D.	
E	Name the structure labelled E.	

Case 4.18

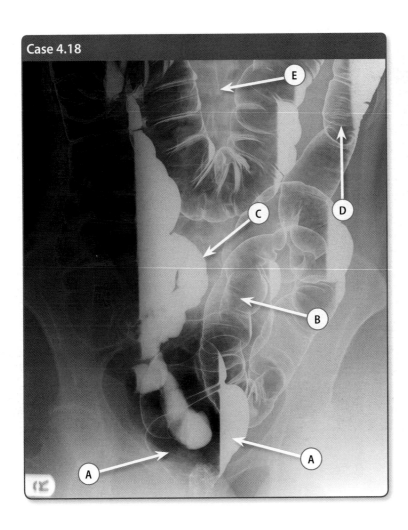

Case 4.18

QUESTION		WRITE YOUR ANSWER HERE
A	Name the structure labelled A.	
B	Name the structure labelled B.	
C	Name the structure labelled C.	
D	Name the structure labelled D.	
E	Name the structure labelled E.	

Case 4.19

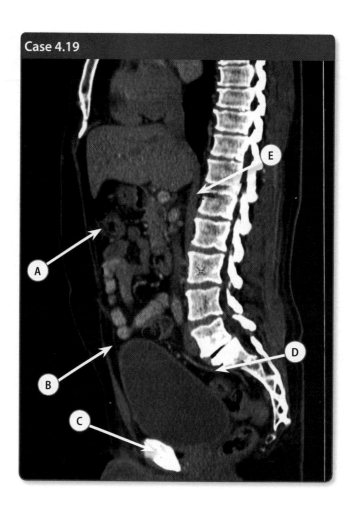

Case 4.19

QUESTION		WRITE YOUR ANSWER HERE
A	Name the structure labelled A.	
B	Name the structure labelled B.	
C	Name the structure labelled C.	
D	Name the structure labelled D.	
E	Name the structure labelled E.	

Case 4.20

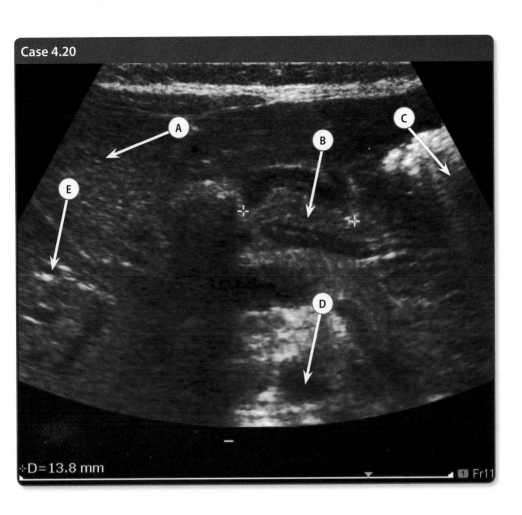

÷D=13.8 mm　　Fr11

Case 4.20

QUESTION		WRITE YOUR ANSWER HERE
A	Name the structure labelled A.	
B	Name the structure labelled B.	
C	Name the structure labelled C.	
D	Name the structure labelled D.	
E	Name the structure labelled E.	

Answers

Case 4.1

A Right trapezoid

B Right hook of hamate

C Right capitate

D Styloid process of right ulna

E Distal right radio-ulnar joint

The eight carpal bones form the proximal and distal carpal rows of the wrist and include: the scaphoid, lunate, triquetral, pisiform, trapezium, trapezoid, capitate and hamate.

An easy mnemonic to remember: **S**cared **L**overs **T**ry **P**ositions **T**hat **T**hey **C**annot **H**andle.

The scaphoid articulates with the radius and is therefore a lateral structure.

The trapezium rhymes with thumb ('the thumb swings on trapezium') allowing easy differentiation from the adjacent trapezoid.

The medially situated hamate can be easily identified due to its characteristic 'Hook'.

Case 4.2

A Trachea

B Azygos lobe

C Azygos fissure

D Azygos vein

E Right scapula

The azygos fissure/lobe is a normal anatomical variant seen in up to 0.4% of chest radiographs and 1% of anatomical specimens. This occurs when one of the precursors of the azygos vein fails to migrate over the apex of the right lung, leading to a mesentery-like fold of pleura, containing two layers of parietal and two of visceral pleura, at the bottom of which lies the azygos vein.

Case 4.3

A Fornix

B Massa intermedia

C Mamillary body

D Pineal gland

E Quadrigeminal (tectal) plate

The pineal gland (shaped like a pine cone, hence its name) is an ovoid structure situated in the posterior wall of the third ventricle, between the two superior colliculi, superior to the quadrigeminal (tectal) plate and anterior to the posterior commissure. Together with the thalamus, hypothalamus and habenula, it is part of the diencephalon.

Pineal gland calcification is present in almost 100% of the adult population.

Case 4.4

A Urinary bladder

B Endometrium

C Myometrium

D Vaginal canal

E 15 mm

The uterus lies posterior to the bladder and anterior to the rectum, usually in an anteflexed and anteverted position. The endometrium has a characteristic trilaminar appearance and may be up to 15 mm thick in women of childbearing age. Following menopause, the endometrium atrophies and should measure less than 5 mm.

Case 4.5

A Right long head of biceps femoris muscle

B Left gracilis muscle

C Left vastus lateralis muscle

D Right rectus femoris muscle

E Left semimembranosus muscle

The anatomy of the thigh is divided into compartments which are bounded by fascial planes. A brief description of the contents of each compartment is provided below.

Anterior

- Iliotibial tract, tensor fascia lata muscle, quadriceps muscles, sartorius muscle

Medial

- Gracilis muscle, adductor muscles

Posterior

- Hamstring muscles, short head of biceps femoris muscle, sciatic nerve.

Case 4.6

A Nasal septum

B Hard palate

C Left temporomandibular joint

D Pulp cavity of second left lower molar tooth

E Crown of left lower lateral incisor

The dental orthopantomogram (OPG) is acquired by synchronous rotation of the X-ray tube and X-ray detector around the patient's head and is a two-dimensional view of the whole mandible and maxilla. The appearances may be a bit confusing – note that the cervical spine is on each side of the mandible.

There are 32 permanent teeth occupying alveoli in the mandible and maxilla. On each side of the upper and lower jaw there are eight teeth, as illustrated in **Table 4.1**.

Table 4.1 Permanent dentition in the right upper jaw							
Molars			Pre-molars		Canine	Incisors	
3rd	2nd	1st	2nd	1st	Solitary	Lateral	Medial

Case 4.7

A Pulmonary artery

B Right coronary artery

C Left atrium

D Oesophagus

E Xiphoid process or xiphisternum

The right coronary artery is seen to arise from the anterior aortic cusp. On sagittal images, the left atrium is the most posterior chamber. The ascending aorta is anterior to this. Density of contrast is higher in the aorta and the right coronary artery as this is timed as a CT coronary angiogram.

Case 4.8

A Sacrum

B Iliopectineal line

C Uterine cavity

D Lumen of left fallopian tube

E Left sacroiliac joint

Hystosalpingography requires the uterine cavity to be filled with contrast by retrograde catheter injection. It is commonly performed to assess the patency of the fallopian tubes. Similar appearances can be obtained with water and utilising a heavy T2-weighted MRI sequence. Free spillage of contrast into the peritoneal cavity confirms tubal patency.

The uterus is located extraperitoneally between the rectum and the bladder. In 90% of the population, the uterus lies in an anteverted and anteflexed position. Retroversion and retroflexion are normal variations in the remaining 10%. The broad ligament, a peritoneal fold, envelops the anterior uterus and attaches the lateral walls of the organ to the pelvis.

Case 4.9

A Sphenoid sinus

B Superficial lobe of the left parotid gland

C Epiglottis

D Right palatine tonsil

E Right medial pterygoid muscle

The pharynx is divided into three levels – the nasopharynx, oropharynx and hypopharynx – in accordance with its communication with the nasal, oral and laryngeal cavities respectively.

The pharyngeal mucosal space, as delineated in **Figure 4.1,** is a fascial space which surrounds the pharynx and contains the pharyngeal constrictor muscles, the extrinsic muscles of the pharynx and lymphoid tissue (the adenoids and tonsils).

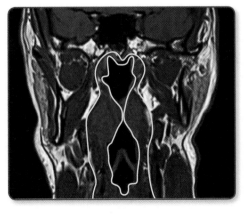

Figure 4.1 Coronal T1-weighted MRI illustrating the pharyngeal mucosal space.

Case 4.10

A Loop of a pigtail catheter in the distal aorta

B Kidney (transplanted)

C Left common iliac artery

D Right internal iliac artery

E Left lumbar artery

Kidneys tend to be transplanted within the pelvis to enable excision of short donor pedicles of artery, vein and ureter. The high vascularity within the renal capillary bed causes a characteristic blush when contrast is injected.

Case 4.11

A Common hepatic duct

B Common bile duct

C Pancreatic duct

D Duodenum (third part)

E Gallbladder

The commonest anatomical form of the biliary system is depicted in this example. (A) shows the common hepatic duct formed by the right and left hepatic ducts. The cystic duct joins the common hepatic duct to form the common bile duct which drains into the second part of the duodenum. The pancreatic duct is also demonstrated and is seen draining into the ampulla.

Variant anatomy is commonly encountered, with several possible variants in the intrahepatic and extrahepatic biliary tree.

Case 4.12

A Right transverse process of C7

B Spinous process of T2

C Right pedicle of T7

D Right hemidiaphragm

E Azygos fissure

The azygos fissure is the most common accessory fissure visible on chest radiography (seen in approximately 1–2%). The azygos vein runs in the most medial aspect of the fissure, surrounded by both parietal and visceral pleura.

A vertebra seen on an anteroposterior radiograph can be thought of as an owl: the spinous process corresponding to the beak, the pedicles representing eyes. The 'winking owl' sign is an important indication of pedicular destruction.

Case 4.13

A Right sylvian fissure (lateral sulcus)

B Third ventricle

C Quadrigeminal cistern

D Left superior colliculus of midbrain

E Falx cerebri

The superior midbrain colliculi lie anterior to the quadrigeminal cistern, and on the axial image are shaped like a 'baby's bottom'. The shape of CSF spaces at this level resembles a 'smiling face', as illustrated in **Figure 4.2**.

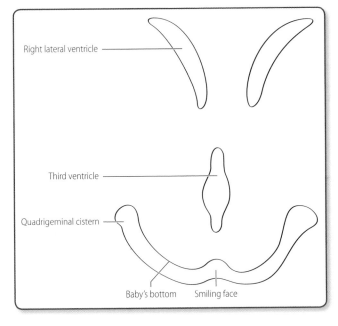

Right lateral ventricle

Third ventricle

Quadrigeminal cistern

Baby's bottom   Smiling face

Figure 4.2 'Smiling face' – schematic illustration of the CSF relationships at the level of the quadrigeminal plate.

Case 4.14

A Right radial head ossification centre

B Right capitulum ossification centre

C Right olecranon fossa

D Right medial epicondyle ossification centre

E Right trochlea ossification centre

Knowledge of the various ossification centres around the elbow joint is important in the assessment of paediatric upper limb trauma.

The mnemonic CRITOL (1-3-5-7-9-11) can be used to remember the order in which ossification centres usually appear: Capitulum (approximately 1 year of age); Radial head (approximately 3 years of age and seen here as a tiny calcific density); Internal (medial) epicondyle (5 years of age); Trochlea (7 years of age); Olecranon (9 years of age and more readily appreciated on a lateral view); and Lateral epicondyle (11 years of age). Fusion is normally complete by the age of 17.

Case 4.15

A Right hepatic vein

B Right renal vein

C Origin of superior mesenteric artery

D Stomach

E Spleen

The inferior vena cava (IVC) most commonly lies to the right of the aorta, although variations of this do exist, e.g. a left IVC draining into the left renal vein.

The coeliac axis and superior mesenteric artery (SMA) are anterior branches of the aorta and arise at the levels of T12 and L1 respectively.

Case 4.16

A Coccyx

B Acetabulum

C Iliac crest

D Superior articular process of L5

E Facet joint between L3 and L4

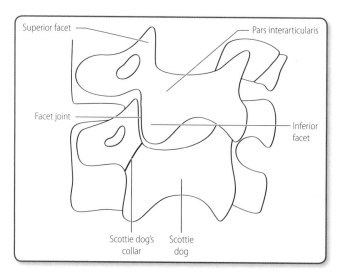

Figure 4.3 Scottie dog's collar is the appearance of a defect in the pars interarticularis.

Coned lateral radiographs of the lumbosacral junction are commonly obtained to assess for spondylolysis and spondylolisthesis. Spondylolysis involves a fracture of the pars interarticularis – the part of a vertebra that lies between its superior and inferior articular facets. On an oblique view, this can be seen as a 'collar' through the neck of a 'Scottie dog' as shown in **Figure 4.3**. Spondylolisthesis describes the vertebral displacement that may occur as a result of spondylolysis.

Case 4.17

A Base of first metatarsal (great toe)

B Dome of talus

C Medial cuneiform

D Talonavicular joint

E Tibialis posterior tendon

One of the most difficult parts of the examination is being shown an image like the one in this case and having to orientate yourself with the information demonstrated on strictly one slice.

This sagittal image has several clues to indicate that the slice is taken through the medial aspect of the ankle and foot. The distal tibia is evident, as are the medial flexor tendons of the ankle – this should guide you to the location being medial. Remember that the talus is located superomedial to the calcaneum, just as the talonavicular joint is relative to the calcaneocuboidal articulation.

Case 4.18

A Rectum

B Sigmoid colon

C Terminal ileum

D Descending colon

E Spinous process

On barium enema examinations, retrograde filling of the terminal ileum (as shown here) and/or the vermiform appendix should be specifically examined for as this confirms that contrast has reached the caecum. Visualised bones should always be scrutinised, as normal osseous structures (e.g. pedicles and spinous processes) may mimic bowel pathologies if projected over the colon.

Case 4.19

    A Transverse colon

    B Peritoneal reflection

    C Right pubis

    D Superior rectal artery

    E Inferior vena cava (IVC)

Orientation of abdominal and pelvic structures in the sagittal plane is easier when you can recognise important anatomical landmarks. The IVC may serve as a good landmark when seen running anterior to the vertebral column and traversing the liver just before crossing the diaphragm to drain into the right atrium.

The superior rectal artery, a branch of the inferior mesenteric artery (IMA), can be identified coursing anteriorly to the sacrum to supply the rectum.

Case 4.20

    A Liver

    B Pylorus

    C Gastric antrum

    D Abdominal aorta

    E Branch of right portal vein

Ultrasound is the imaging modality of choice when evaluating suspected infantile hypertrophic pyloric stenosis. Normally, the pylorus muscle should not exceed 3 mm in thickness and the pylorus should be no more than 17 mm in length, although this is somewhat contingent on the size of the infant. The muscular layers of the pylorus are hypoechoic with hyperechoity of the mucosa. The stomach itself may appear as a solid structure on ultrasound if distended with milk curd.

Portal vein branches can be differentiated from intrahepatic bile ducts by their increased reflectivity, as shown in this case.

Chapter 5

Mock paper 5

20 cases to be answered in 75 minutes

Case 5.1

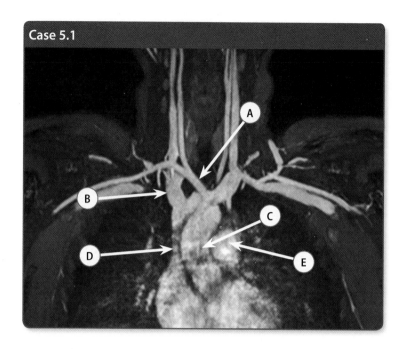

Case 5.1

QUESTION		WRITE YOUR ANSWER HERE
A	Name the structure labelled A.	
B	Name the structure labelled B.	
C	Name the structure labelled C.	
D	Name the structure labelled D.	
E	Name the structure labelled E.	

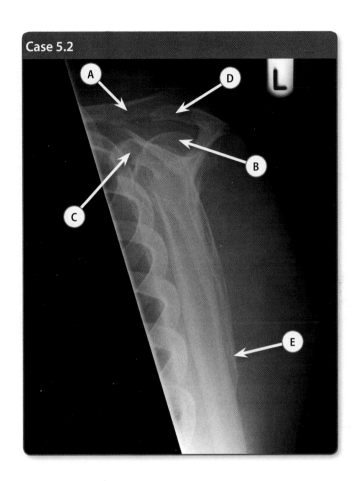

Case 5.2

Case 5.2		
QUESTION		**WRITE YOUR ANSWER HERE**
A	Name the structure labelled A.	
B	Name the structure labelled B.	
C	Name the structure labelled C.	
D	Name the structure labelled D.	
E	Name the structure labelled E.	

Case 5.3

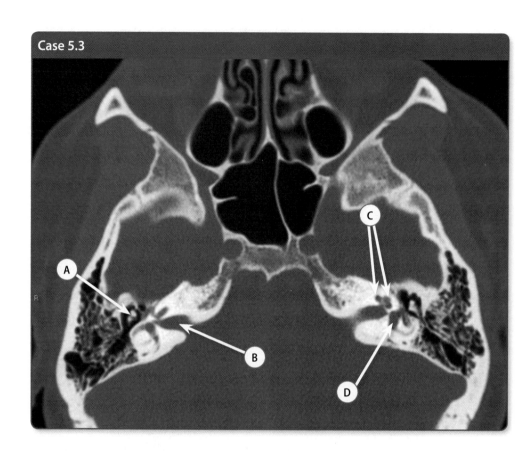

Case 5.3

QUESTION		WRITE YOUR ANSWER HERE
A	Name the joint labelled A.	
B	Name the structure labelled B.	
C	Name the structure labelled C.	
D	Name the structure labelled D.	
E	Which cranial nerve passes through the middle ear cavity?	

Case 5.4

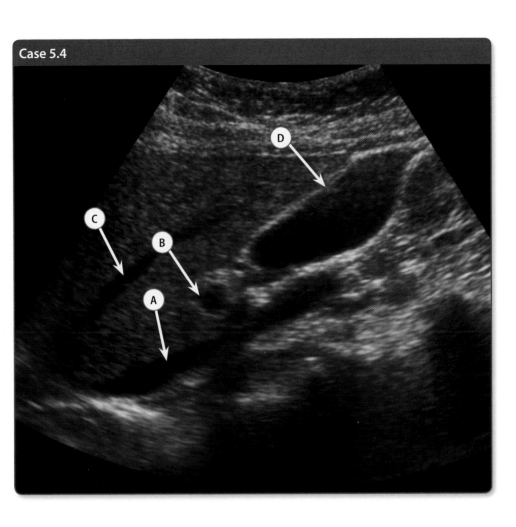

Case 5.4

QUESTION		WRITE YOUR ANSWER HERE
A	Name the structure labelled A.	
B	Name the structure labelled B.	
C	Name the structure labelled C	
D	Name the structure labelled D.	
E	What is the normal upper limit of wall thickness of the gallbladder?	

Case 5.5

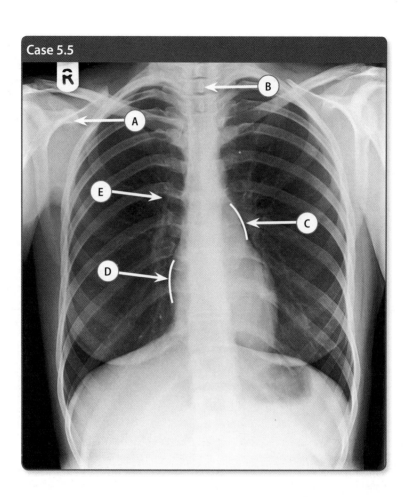

Case 5.5

QUESTION		WRITE YOUR ANSWER HERE
A	Name the structure labelled A.	
B	Name the structure labelled B.	
C	Name the structure labelled C (outlined by a line).	
D	Name the structure labelled D (outlined by a line).	
E	Name the lucent structure labelled E.	

Case 5.6

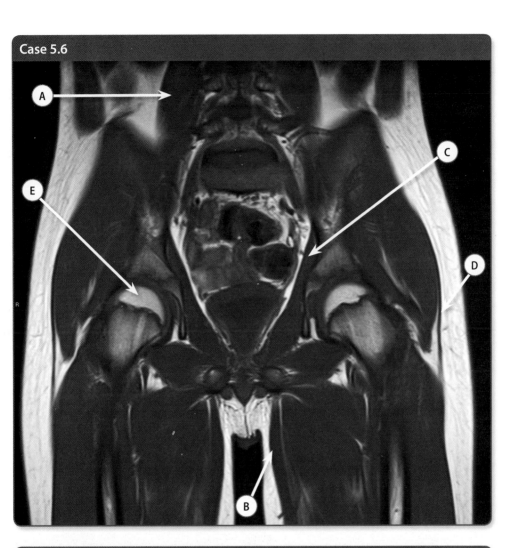

Case 5.6

QUESTION		WRITE YOUR ANSWER HERE
A	Name the tendinous insertion site for the structure labelled A.	
B	Name the origin of the structure labelled B.	
C	Name the structure labelled C.	
D	Name the structure labelled D.	
E	Name the structure labelled E.	

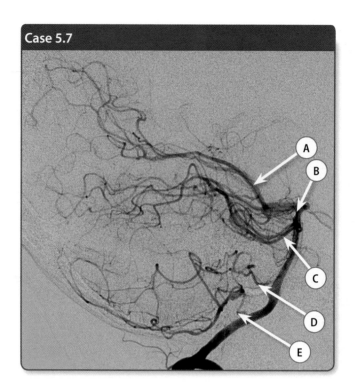

Case 5.7

Case 5.7

QUESTION		WRITE YOUR ANSWER HERE
A	Name the structure labelled A.	
B	Name the structure labelled B.	
C	Name the structure labelled C.	
D	Name the structure labelled D.	
E	Name the structure labelled E.	

Case 5.8

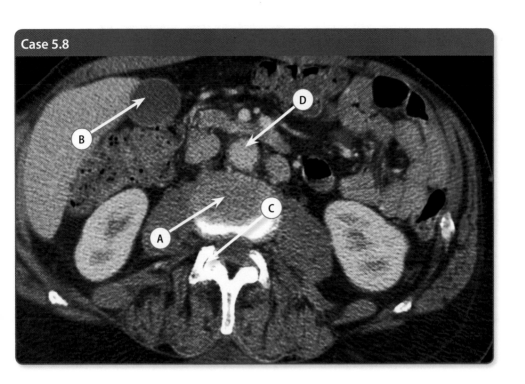

Case 5.8

QUESTION		WRITE YOUR ANSWER HERE
A	Name the structure labelled A.	
B	Name the structure labelled B.	
C	Name the structure labelled C.	
D	Name the structure labelled D.	
E	Which anatomical variant is present on this image?	

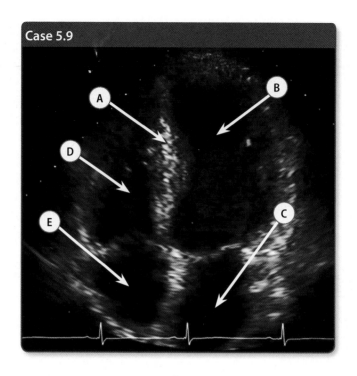

Case 5.9

QUESTION		WRITE YOUR ANSWER HERE
A	Name the structure labelled A.	
B	Name the chamber labelled B.	
C	Name the chamber labelled C.	
D	Name the chamber labelled D.	
E	Name the chamber labelled E.	

Case 5.10

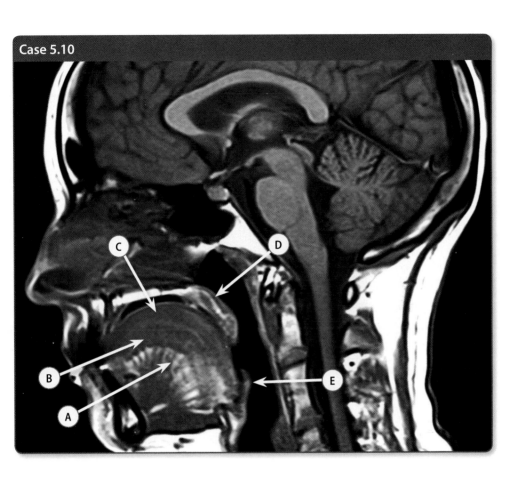

Case 5.10

QUESTION		WRITE YOUR ANSWER HERE
A	Name the structure labelled A.	
B	Name the structure labelled B.	
C	Name the structure labelled C.	
D	Name the structure labelled D.	
E	Name the structure labelled E.	

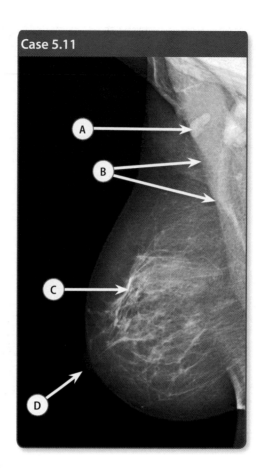

Case 5.11

Case 5.11

QUESTION		WRITE YOUR ANSWER HERE
A	Name the structure labelled A.	
B	What muscle is labelled B?	
C	Name the structure labelled C.	
D	Name the structure labelled D.	
E	What is the tissue behind the nipple called?	

Case 5.12

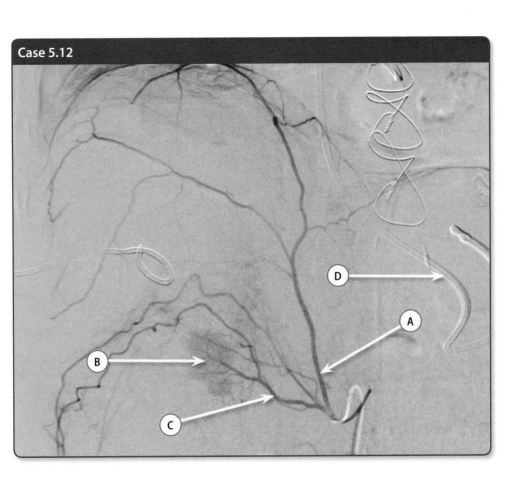

Case 5.12

QUESTION		WRITE YOUR ANSWER HERE
A	Name the structure labelled A.	
B	Name the structure labelled B.	
C	Name the structure labelled C.	
D	Name the tube labelled D.	
E	How many arteries usually supply the adrenal gland?	

Case 5.13

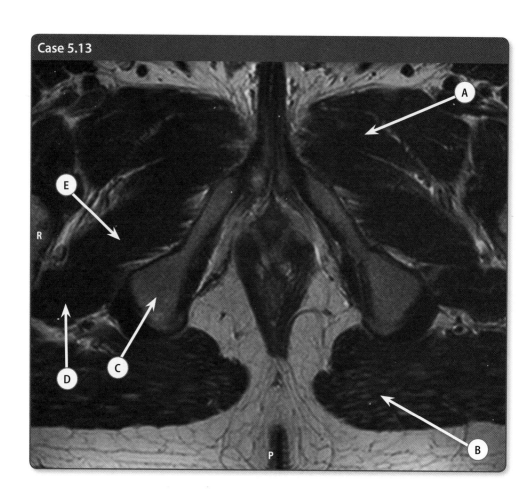

Case 5.13

QUESTION		WRITE YOUR ANSWER HERE
A	Name the structure labelled A.	
B	Name the structure labelled B.	
C	Name the structure labelled C.	
D	Name the structure labelled D.	
E	Name the structure labelled E.	

Case 5.14

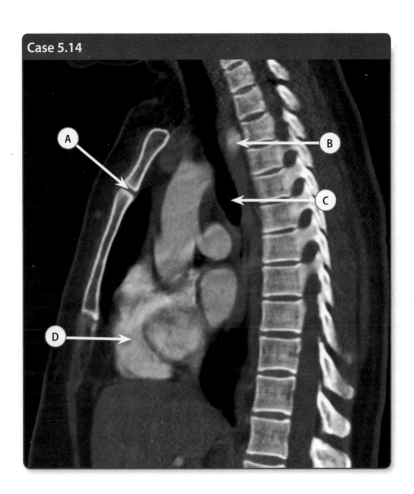

Case 5.14

QUESTION		WRITE YOUR ANSWER HERE
A	Name the structure labelled A.	
B	Name the structure labelled B.	
C	Name the structure labelled C.	
D	Name the chamber labelled D.	
E	What is the focal dilatation of the aorta called (caused by the anatomical variant present)?	

Case 5.15

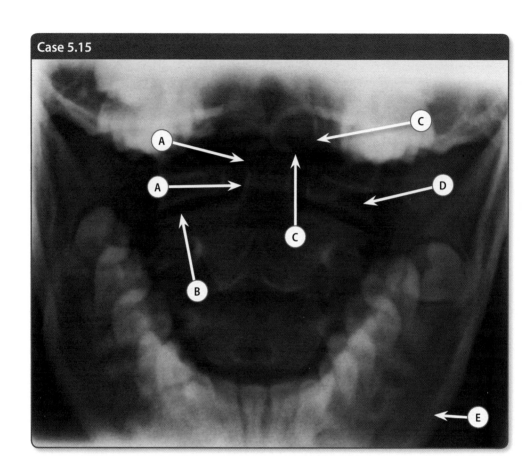

Case 5.15

QUESTION		WRITE YOUR ANSWER HERE
A	Name the structure labelled A.	
B	Name the joint labelled B.	
C	Name the structure labelled C.	
D	Name the structure labelled D.	
E	Name the structure labelled E.	

Case 5.16

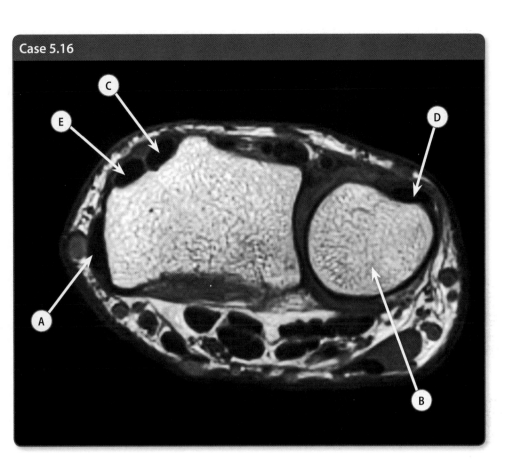

Case 5.16

QUESTION		WRITE YOUR ANSWER HERE
A	Name the structure labelled A.	
B	Name the structure labelled B.	
C	Name the structure labelled C.	
D	Name the structure labelled D.	
E	Name the structure labelled E.	

Case 5.17

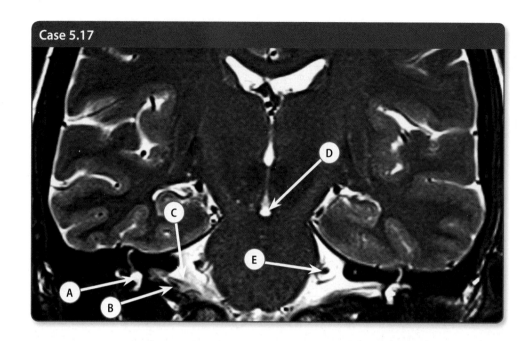

Case 5.17

QUESTION		WRITE YOUR ANSWER HERE
A	Name the structure labelled A.	
B	Name the structure labelled B.	
C	Name the structure labelled C.	
D	Name the structure labelled D.	
E	Name the structure labelled E.	

Case 5.18

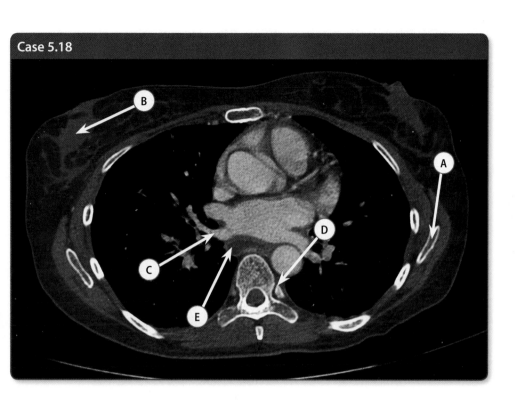

Case 5.18

QUESTION		WRITE YOUR ANSWER HERE
A	Name the structure labelled A.	
B	Name the structure labelled B.	
C	Name the structure labelled C.	
D	Name the joint labelled D.	
E	Name the structure labelled E.	

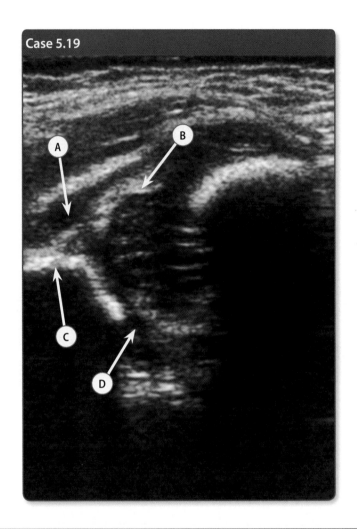

Case 5.19

Case 5.19	
QUESTION	**WRITE YOUR ANSWER HERE**
A	Name the structure labelled A.	
B	Name the structure labelled B.	
C	Name the structure labelled C.	
D	Name the structure labelled D.	
E	What is the name of the angle used to assess the acetabular depth?	

Case 5.20

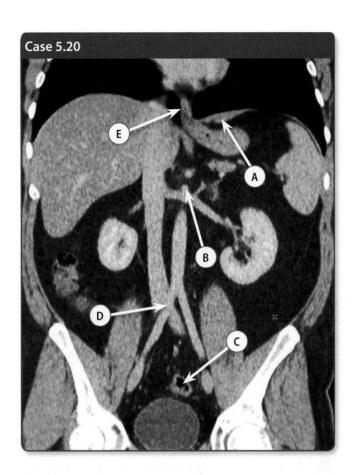

Case 5.20

QUESTION		WRITE YOUR ANSWER HERE
A	Name the structure labelled A.	
B	Name the structure labelled B.	
C	Name the structure labelled C.	
D	Name the structure labelled D.	
E	Name the structure labelled E.	

Answers

Case 5.1

A Brachiocephalic trunk/innominate artery

B Right brachiocephalic vein

C Ascending aorta

D Superior vena cava

E Pulmonary trunk/main pulmonary artery

This coronal maximum intensity projection (MIP) slab demonstrates the arterial and venous anatomy of the chest and neck.

The brachiocephalic veins combine to form the superior vena cava (SVC). The internal jugular and the subclavian veins unite to form the brachiocephalic veins.

This is the most common anatomical configuration of the aortic arch, with the brachiocephalic trunk, left common carotid and left subclavian artery emerging from the arch from proximal to distal.

Case 5.2

A Distal left clavicle

B Head of left humerus

C Coracoid process of left scapula

D Acromion of left scapula

E Blade of left scapula

The lateral scapular view, also known as the 'Y' view, may be difficult to interpret. However, orientating yourself with simple landmarks will allow you to easily put all the pieces of the puzzle together.

Key landmarks:

- The distal clavicle articulates with the acromion at the acromioclavicular (AC) joint
- The coracoid process points anteriorly (hence the humeral head is visualised beneath the coracoid in an anterior glenohumeral dislocation)
- The spine of the scapula is a horizontal bony boundary between the supraspinatus and infraspinatus muscles.

Case 5.3

A Right incudomalleolar joint

B Right internal auditory canal

C Left cochlea

D Left vestibulum

E Facial nerve (VII)

This high resolution CT depicts the petrous portion of the temporal bone with great precision. The structures of the middle ear have very characteristic names, of which a little imagination and Latin will help:

- **Cochlea** – Latin for 'snail shell' as it is coiled.
- **Vestibulum** – Latin for 'entrance hall' which is indeed the reception for the inner ear
- **Labyrinth** – derived from Greek mythology and representing a complicated maze-like structure. You find its analogy in the inner ear labyrinth, with a system of passages comprising cochlea, vestibulum and three semicircular canals
- **Auditory ossicles** – malleus (Latin for hammer), incus (anvil-shaped) and stapes (stirrup-shaped) articulate with each other in that order. The facial nerve crosses the middle ear cavity, helping create an easy to remember mnemonic:

  MISS – Malleus-Incus-Stapes-Seventh nerve
  Incus and malleus articulate with each other at the incudomalleolar joint, forming the characteristic 'ice cream cone' shape which is best appreciated on axial CT.

Case 5.4

A Inferior vena cava

B Portal vein

C Hepatic vein

D Gallbladder

E 3 mm

This image shows the gallbladder in longitudinal section, the fundus evident near the top of the image and the neck in the middle of the image. One of the three hepatic veins is seen coursing towards the inferior vena cava, usually joining it just before the inferior vena cava reaches the right atrium.

Case 5.5

A Coracoid process of the right scapula

B Spinous process of T2

C Left atrial appendage

D Lateral border of the right atrium

E Right upper lobe segmental bronchus (end on)

In the cardiac silhouette, it is important to know the borders of the heart and the chambers which form them. The lower right heart border is formed by the right atrium and the upper right silhouette created by the superior vena cava.

The bulge of the left atrial appendage contributes to the left heart border superiorly, with the inferior left heart border formed by the left ventricle.

The right ventricle forms most of the inferior border of the heart.

Case 5.6

A Lesser trochanter of right femur

B Left inferior pubic ramus

C Left obturator internus muscle

D Left iliotibial band

E Right capital femoral epiphysis

Psoas major

- Origin – transverse processes of the L1–L5 vertebrae and lateral surfaces of the T12–L4 vertebrae
- Insertion – common iliopsoas insertion into the lesser trochanter of proximal femur.

Gracilis

- Origin – inferior pubic ramus, arising from aponeurosis
- Insertion – pes anserinus (proximal medial tibia).

Obturator internus

- Origin – ischiopubic rami
- Insertion – Trochanteric fossa, greater trochanter of femur.

The iliotibial band is a fibrous enforcement of the fascia lata and the insertion site of gluteus maximus and tensor fascia lata.

Case 5.7

A Posterior cerebral artery

B Basilar tip

C Superior cerebellar artery

D Anterior inferior cerebellar artery

E Posterior inferior cerebellar artery

The vertebrobasilar circulation resembles a 'tree' on DSA angiography. On the frontal projection, it looks like a 'tree on a windless day' (see Figure 8.1), whereas on the lateral projection it is shaped like a 'tree on a windy day' (**Figure 5.1**).

Two vertebral arteries join to form a single basilar artery (BA) at the pontomedullary junction. The posterior inferior cerebral artery (PICA) – the largest branch of the vertebral artery – arises distally, just before the vertebral confluence. The BA gives off

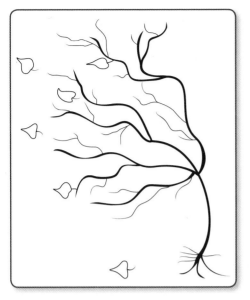

Figure 5.1 'Tree on a windy day' resembling the vertebrobasilar circulation on the lateral DSA angiography.

two large branches on each side: the anterior inferior (AICA) and superior cerebellar arteries (SCA).

The posterior cerebral arteries (PCA) are terminal branches of the basilar artery.

Case 5.8

A Intervertebral disc

B Gallbladder

C Right facet joint

D Abdominal aorta

E Double inferior vena cava

The double inferior vena cava (IVC) has a prevalence of 0.2–3.0% and is a result of the persistence of both sacrocardinal veins. The left IVC typically drains into the left renal vein, although numerous other variations have been described.

The aorta was purposely labelled to focus attention on the rather symmetrical coursing of the IVC on either side of it. The exam will not necessarily point out what variant is present and it will be up to you to identify and correctly label it.

The following venous variants may show up:

- Double IVC
- Retroaortic left renal vein
- Left IVC
- Azygous continuation of the IVC (absence of the hepatic segment of the IVC with azygous continuation)
- Circumaortic left renal vein

Case 5.9

    A Interventricular septum

    B Left ventricle

    C Left atrium

    D Right ventricle

    E Right atrium

This is an apical four-chamber view echocardiogram. The transducer is placed close to the palpated apex beat of the heart, on the left side of the chest. The left ventricle is usually the larger of the two chambers and is thick walled. The atria are noted at the base of the view.

In this view, the left ventricle is on the top right with the left atrium opening into it through the mitral valve, and the right ventricle is on the left side with the right atrium opening into it through the tricuspid valve. This view is useful to compare the thickness of the left and right ventricular walls and to determine whether or not a pericardial effusion is present.

Case 5.10

    A Genioglossus muscle

    B Intrinsic transverse muscle of the tongue

    C Intrinsic longitudinal muscle of the tongue

    D Soft palate

    E Epiglottis

The tongue forms part of the floor of the mouth. It comprises intrinsic muscles which lie in three planes: transverse, longitudinal and vertical. The muscles are separated by fat planes which are important landmarks on imaging. The tongue is supported by three extrinsic muscles – styloglossus, genioglossus and hypoglossus – with the genioglossus muscle, running between the tongue and the posterior aspect of the mandible, being the largest.

Case 5.11

    A Right axillary lymph node

    B Right pectoralis major muscle

    C Right intramammary blood vessels

    D Right nipple

    E Retroareolar tissue

The pectoralis major muscle is seen at the base of the breast. The axillary tail of the breast and accessory breast tissue may be seen in the axilla. Normal anatomical structures such as intramammary blood vessels and lymph nodes may also be seen on mammograms. The other conventional mammographic view is the craniocaudal view which is almost orthogonal to the mediolateral oblique (MLO) view.

Case 5.12

A Right inferior phrenic artery

B Right adrenal gland

C Right superior suprarenal artery

D Nasogastric tube

E Three

The inferior phrenic arteries arise from abdominal aorta close to the origin of the coeliac axis. The superior suprarenal artery can arise from this and supplies the adrenal gland.

The adrenal gland also derives blood supply from the middle suprarenal artery (branch of abdominal aorta) and the inferior suprarenal artery, which is a branch of the renal artery.

Case 5.13

A Left adductor longus muscle

B Left gluteus maximus muscle

C Right ischium

D Right quadratus femoris muscle

E Right adductor magnus muscle

The three adductor muscles (magnus, longus and brevis) have a common origin site from the external surface of the pubic bone. The muscle surrounding the anus is the puborectalis which is the inferior part of the levator ani muscles. The fat-filled spaces immediately lateral to the anal complex are the ischioanal fossae. These contain small dark serpiginous structures anteriorly (as seen on this image) which are the inferior neurovascular bundles.

Case 5.14

A Manubriosternal joint

B Aberrant right subclavian artery

C Trachea

D Right ventricle

E Diverticulum of Kommerell

The course of an aberrant right subclavian artery is often retro-oesophageal and it will cause a posterior indentation of the oesophagus on a barium swallow.

On this sagittal view, orientation is important. The right ventricle is the most anterior chamber of the heart in the midline sagittal view. The left ventricle can be seen appearing into view just posterior to this.

Case 5.15

A Odontoid peg

B Right atlantoaxial joint

C Left central incisor

D Left lateral mass of C1

E Body of the left hemimandible

Peg views of the cervical spine are performed to assess the relative alignment of the lateral masses of C1 (the atlas) to C2 (the axis). The joint between them is the atlantoaxial joint. Detail may be obscured by overlapping teeth and the hard palate, which can also mimic fracture lines.

Case 5.16

A Abductor pollicis longus tendon or (other acceptable answer) extensor pollicis brevis tendon

B Distal ulna

C Extensor carpi radialis longus tendon

D Extensor carpi ulnaris tendon

E Extensor carpi radialis brevis tendon

The tendons of the dorsal wrist are separated into six fibro-osseous compartments. They include (from radial to ulnar):

1. Abductor pollicis longus and extensor pollicis brevis tendons

2. Extensor carpi radialis longus and brevis tendons

3. Extensor pollicis longus tendon

4. Extensor digitorum and extensor indicis tendons

5. Extensor digiti minimi tendon

6. Extensor carpi ulnaris tendon – lies within the distal ulnar groove.

The dorsal tubercle of the radius, Lister's tubercle, is a helpful osseous landmark between the extensor carpi radialis tendons (second compartment) and the extensor pollicis longus tendon (third compartment).

Case 5.17

A Right vestibule

B Cochlear branch of the right vestibulocochlear nerve (VIII)

C Right facial nerve (VII)

D Interpeduncular cistern

E Left trigeminal nerve (V)

Four nerves pass through the internal auditory meatus (IAM):

- Facial nerve, and

Three branches of the vestibulocochlear nerve:

- Cochlear nerve
- Superior vestibular branch
- Inferior vestibular branch.

Vestibular nerves occupy the posterior part of the IAM. The facial and cochlear nerves are situated in the anterior portion of the IAM, with the facial nerve running superiorly and the cochlear nerve inferiorly. The following mnemonic is useful for remembering their relative positions, 'Seven up, Coke down':

Seven **up** – Seventh (VII) nerve **superior**

Coke **down** – Cochlear nerve **inferior**

Case 5.18

A Left scapula

B Right breast tissue

C Right inferior pulmonary vein

D Left costovertebral joint

E Oesophagus

There are three aortic sinuses or sinuses of Valsalva: the anterior or right coronary sinus, giving off (as its name suggests) the right coronary artery; the left posterior or left coronary sinus giving off the left coronary artery (seen on this image lying in the fat to the left of the ascending aorta and posterior to the pulmonary trunk); and the right posterior or non-coronary sinus.

The oesophagus on this image contains a small amount of fluid which is a common finding on CT examinations, particularly in older patients, and does not necessarily imply obstruction.

Case 5.19

A Gluteal muscles

B Acetabular labrum

C Ilium

D Gap of triradiate cartilage

E Alpha angle

This is the standard coronal ultrasound view of the infantile hip, undertaken to assess for the presence of instability or dislocation. The alpha angle is used to assess acetabular depth. It is ascertained by drawing a line parallel to the ilium and another line from the edge of the acetabulum through the gap of the triradiate cartilage (the lowest part of the bony acetabulum), and determining the angle between them. This should normally be greater than 60°. The beta angle (used to evaluate the labral prominence) is found between the line parallel to the ilium and another line drawn parallel to the edge of the labrum.

These angles and relevant anatomical landmarks are depicted in **Figure 5.2**.

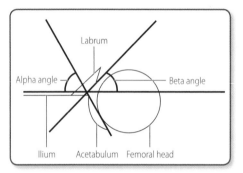

Figure 5.2 Schematic diagram of the infant hip ultrasound.

Case 5.20

A Left hemidiaphragm

B Superior mesenteric artery

C Sigmoid colon

D Right common iliac artery

E Gastro-oesophageal junction

The inferior vena cava (IVC) is the largest abdominal vein which drains blood from the lower limbs and trunk into the right atrium. The IVC runs alongside the vertebral column to the right of the abdominal aorta. It is formed by the confluence of the common iliac veins at the level of L5 and traverses the diaphragm at T8. The main tributaries of the IVC are as follows:

- Hepatic veins (T8 level)
- Inferior phrenic vein (T8)
- Suprarenal vein and renal veins (L1)

- Gonadal vein (L2)
- Lumbar veins (L1)

Note the position of the superior mesenteric artery anterior to the left renal vein. Also note how the right common iliac artery passes anterior to the left common iliac vein.

Chapter 6

Mock paper 6

20 cases to be answered in 75 minutes

Case 6.1

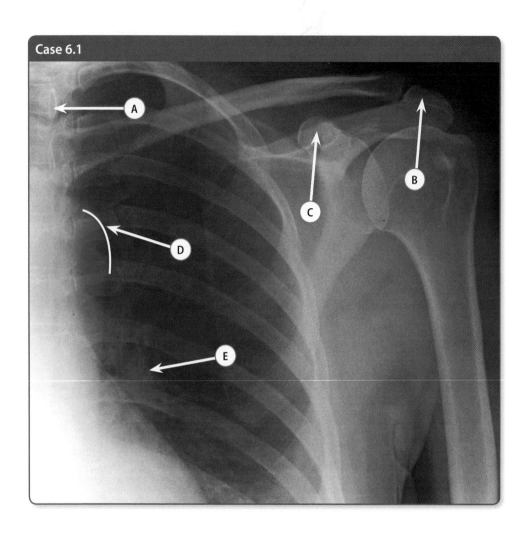

Case 6.1

QUESTION		WRITE YOUR ANSWER HERE
A	Name the structure labelled A.	
B	Name the structure labelled B.	
C	Name the structure labelled C.	
D	Name the structure labelled D.	
E	Name the vascular structure labelled E.	

Case 6.2

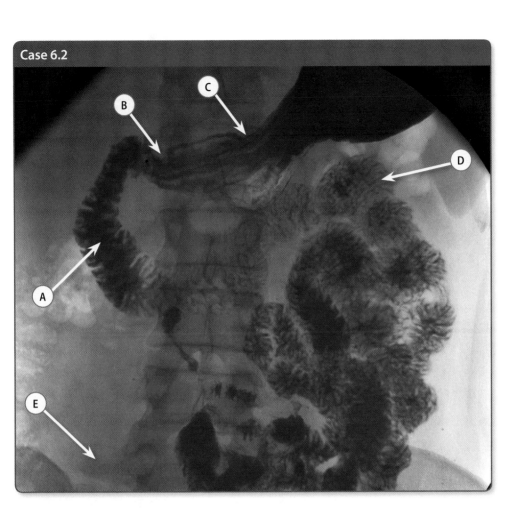

Case 6.2

QUESTION		WRITE YOUR ANSWER HERE
A	Name the structure labelled A.	
B	Name the structure labelled B.	
C	Name the structure labelled C.	
D	Name the structure labelled D.	
E	Name the structure labelled E.	

Case 6.3

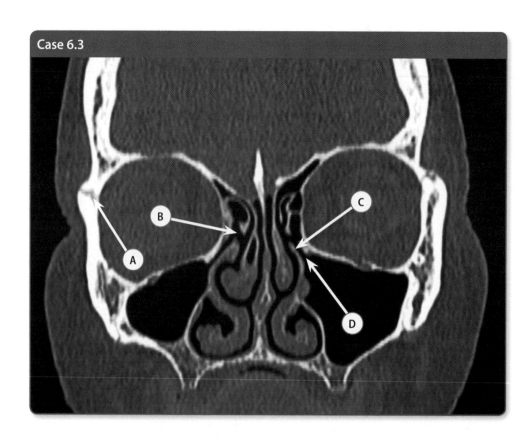

Case 6.3

QUESTION		WRITE YOUR ANSWER HERE
A	Name the structure labelled A.	
B	Name the structure labelled B.	
C	Name the structure labelled C.	
D	Name the structure labelled D.	
E	What is the common final pathway for drainage of the maxillary, frontal and anterior/ middle ethmoid sinuses called?	

Case 6.4

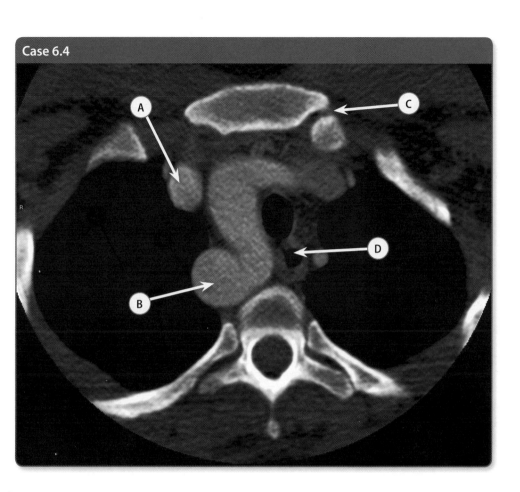

Case 6.4

QUESTION		WRITE YOUR ANSWER HERE
A	Name the structure labelled A.	
B	Name the structure labelled B.	
C	Name the structure labelled C	
D	Name the structure labelled D.	
E	Which anatomical variant is present on this image?	

Case 6.5

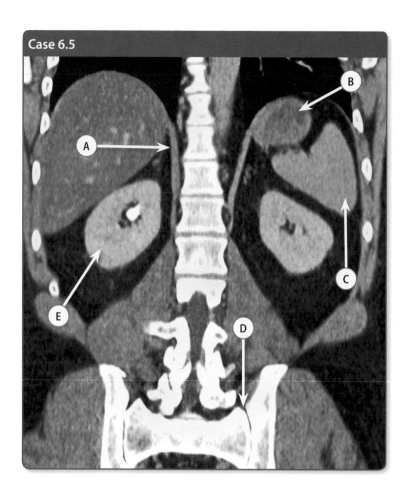

Case 6.5

QUESTION		WRITE YOUR ANSWER HERE
A	Name the structure labelled A.	
B	Name the structure labelled B.	
C	Name the structure labelled C.	
D	Name the joint labelled D.	
E	Name the structure labelled E.	

Case 6.6

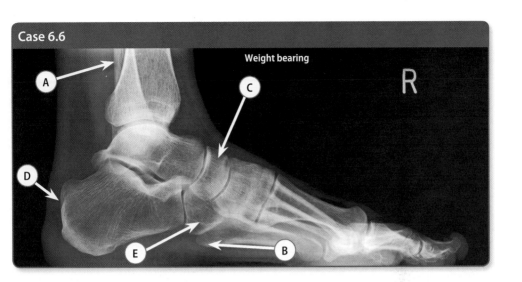

Weight bearing

Case 6.6

QUESTION		WRITE YOUR ANSWER HERE
A	Name the structure labelled A.	
B	Name the structure labelled B.	
C	Name the structure labelled C.	
D	Name the tendon that inserts into the structure labelled D.	
E	Name the structure labelled E.	

Case 6.7

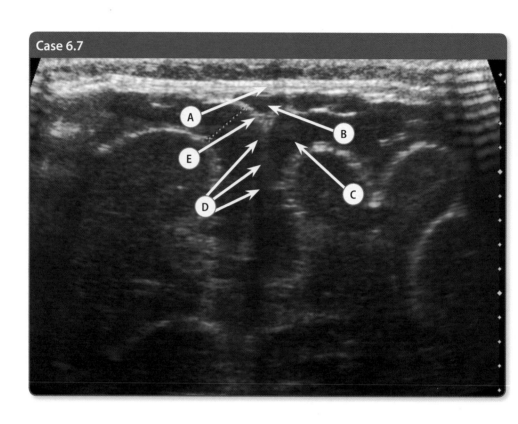

Case 6.7

QUESTION		WRITE YOUR ANSWER HERE
A	Name the structure labelled A.	
B	Name the structure labelled B.	
C	Name the structure labelled C.	
D	Name the structure labelled D.	
E	Name the structure labelled E.	

Case 6.8

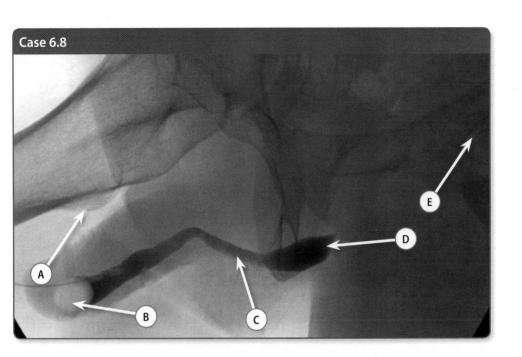

Case 6.8

QUESTION		WRITE YOUR ANSWER HERE
A	Name the structure labelled A.	
B	Name the artificial structure labelled B.	
C	Name the structure labelled C.	
D	Name the joint labelled D.	
E	Name the joint labelled E.	

Case 6.9

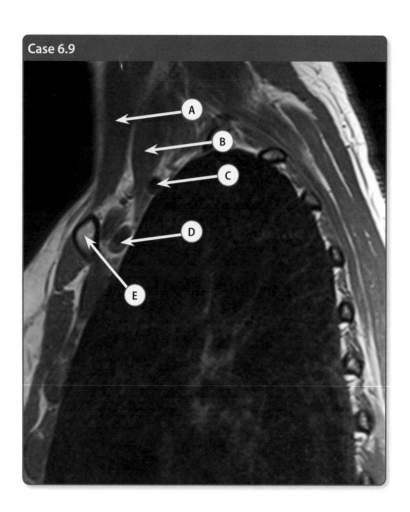

Case 6.9

QUESTION		WRITE YOUR ANSWER HERE
A	Name the structure labelled A.	
B	Name the structure labelled B.	
C	Name the structure labelled C.	
D	Name the structure labelled D.	
E	Name the structure labelled E.	

Case 6.10

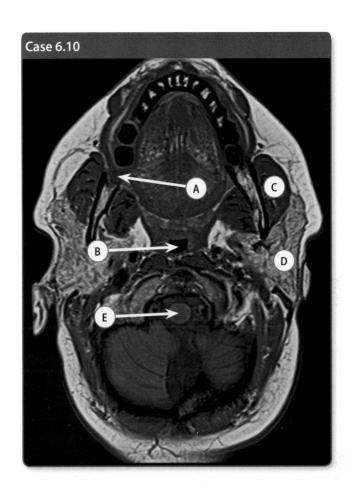

Case 6.10

QUESTION		WRITE YOUR ANSWER HERE
A	Name the structure labelled A.	
B	Name the structure labelled B.	
C	Name the structure labelled C.	
D	Name the structure labelled D.	
E	Name the structure labelled E.	

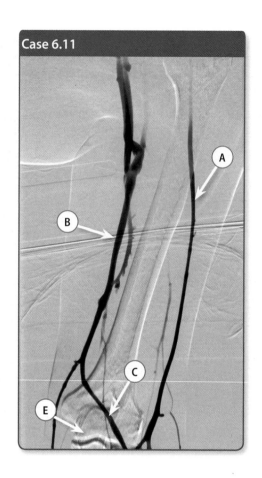

Case 6.11

Case 6.11	
QUESTION	**WRITE YOUR ANSWER HERE**
A Name the structure labelled A.	
B Name the structure labelled B.	
C Name the structure labelled C.	
D What vein is formed by the confluence of the brachial and basilic veins?	
E Name the structure labelled E.	

Case 6.12

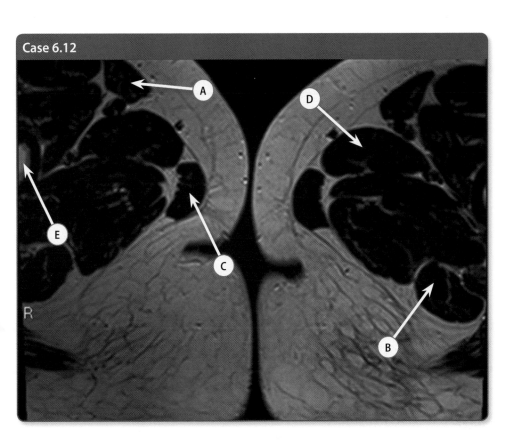

Case 6.12

QUESTION		WRITE YOUR ANSWER HERE
A	What is the origin of the structure labelled A.	
B	Name the structure labelled B.	
C	Name the structure labelled C.	
D	Name the structure labelled D.	
E	Name the structure labelled E.	

Case 6.13

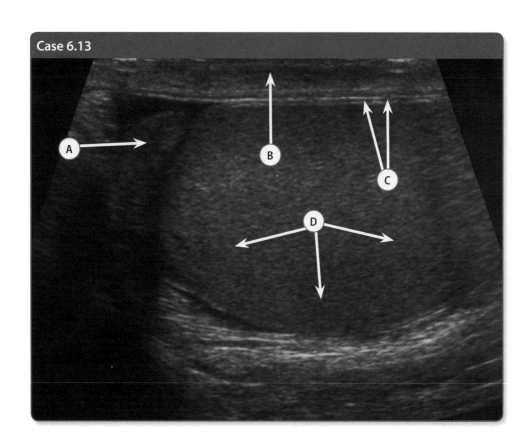

Case 6.13

QUESTION		WRITE YOUR ANSWER HERE
A	Name the structure labelled A.	
B	Name the structure labelled B.	
C	What does the hypoechoic line labelled C correspond to?	
D	Name the structure labelled D.	
E	From where does the left testicular artery arise?	

Case 6.14

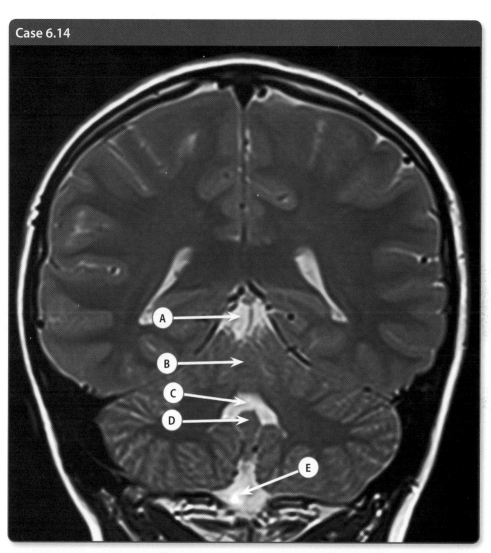

Case 6.14

QUESTION		WRITE YOUR ANSWER HERE
A	Name the structure labelled A.	
B	Name the structure labelled B.	
C	Name the structure labelled C.	
D	Name the structure labelled D.	
E	Name the structure labelled E.	

Case 6.15

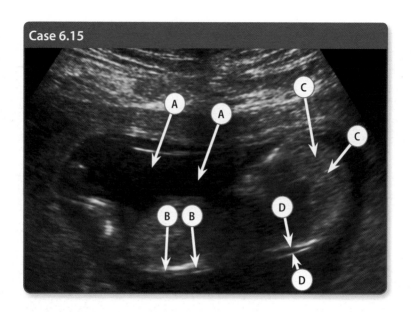

Case 6.15

	QUESTION	WRITE YOUR ANSWER HERE
A	Name the cavity labelled A.	
B	Name the structure labelled B.	
C	Name the structure labelled C.	
D	What measurement is taken between the two 'D' arrows?	
E	What cranial measurement can be used to assess gestational age between 12 and 24 weeks gestation?	

Case 6.16

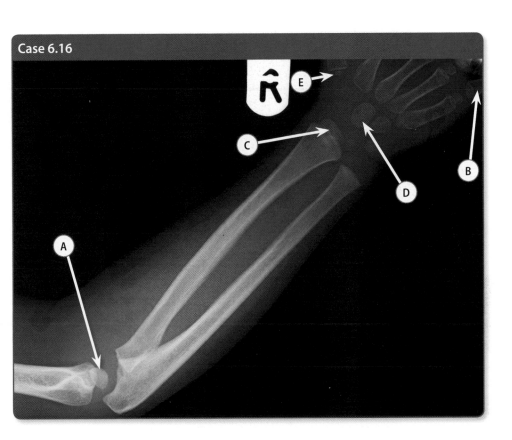

Case 6.16

QUESTION		WRITE YOUR ANSWER HERE
A	Name the structure labelled A.	
B	Name the structure labelled B.	
C	Name the structure labelled C.	
D	Name the structure labelled D.	
E	Name the structure labelled E.	

Case 6.17

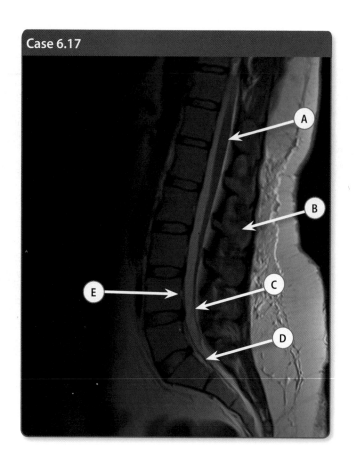

Case 6.17

QUESTION		WRITE YOUR ANSWER HERE
A	Name the structure labelled A.	
B	Name the structure labelled B.	
C	Name the structure labelled C.	
D	Name the structure labelled D.	
E	Name the structure labelled E.	

Case 6.18

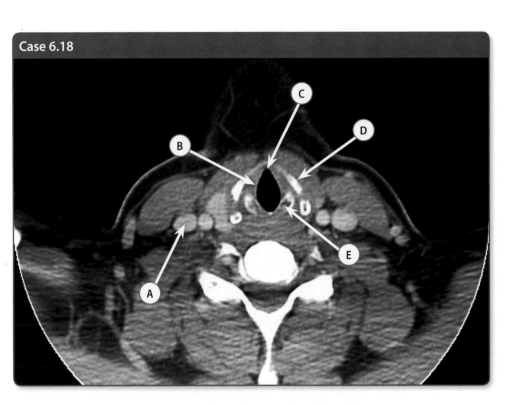

Case 6.18

QUESTION		WRITE YOUR ANSWER HERE
A	Name the structure labelled A.	
B	Name the structure labelled B.	
C	Name the structure labelled C.	
D	Name the structure labelled D.	
E	Name the structure labelled E.	

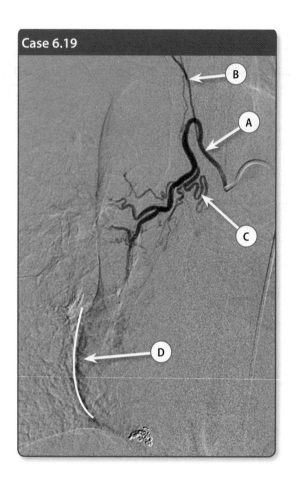

Case 6.19

Case 6.19	
QUESTION	**WRITE YOUR ANSWER HERE**
A Name the structure labelled A.	
B Name the structure labelled B.	
C Name the structure labelled C.	
D Name the structure outlined and labelled D.	
E How many bronchial arteries usually arise from the aorta?	

Case 6.20

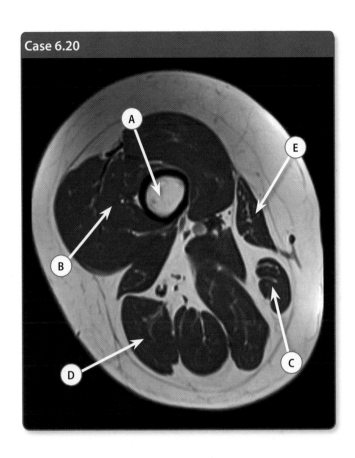

Case 6.20		
QUESTION		**WRITE YOUR ANSWER HERE**
A	Name the structure labelled A.	
B	Name the structure labelled B.	
C	Name the structure labelled C.	
D	Name the structure labelled D.	
E	Name the structure labelled E.	

Answers

Case 6.1

A Spinous process of T2

B Left acromion process

C Left coracoid process

D Arch of aorta (aortic knuckle)

E Left lower lobe pulmonary artery

The three ligaments that attach to the coracoid process are:

1. Coracoclavicular ligament
2. Coracoacromial ligament
3. Coracohumeral ligament.

Case 6.2

A Second part of duodenum

B Pylorus

C Angularis incisura

D Duodenojejunal junction/proximal jejunum (alternative acceptable answer)

E Right L5 transverse process

Blood supply to the proximal duodenum is derived from branches of the coeliac axis (gastroduodenal and superior pancreaticoduodenal arteries). The distal duodenum is supplied by branches of the superior mesenteric artery via the inferior pancreaticoduodenal artery.

The ligament of Treitz marks the duodenojejunal junction and the beginning of the jejunum.

Case 6.3

A Right frontozygomatic suture

B Right ethmoid infundibulum

C Left uncinate process

D Left maxillary sinus ostium

E Ostiomeatal complex

The ostiomeatal complex is a common pathway for the maxillary, frontal and anterior/middle ethmoid sinuses as illustrated in **Figure 6.1**. It consists of:

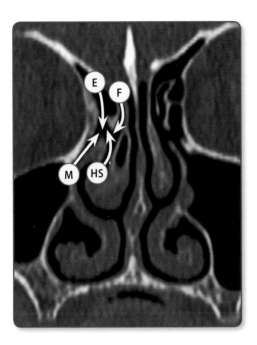

Figure 6.1 The ostiomeatal complex in coronal plane. M, maxillary sinus ostium; E, ethmoid infundibulum; F, frontal recess; HS, hiatus semilunaris.

- **Maxillary sinus ostium** – aperture of the maxillary sinus (M)
- **Ethmoid infundibulum** – opening of the anterior/middle ethmoid cells (E)
- **Frontal recess** – ostium for frontal sinus (F)
- **Hiatus semilunaris (HS)** – a crescentic groove forming a common location of the above openings

Case 6.4

A Superior vena cava

B Descending thoracic aorta

C Left sternoclavicular joint

D Oesophagus

E Right aortic arch

A right-sided aortic arch can be of two types, commonly:

1. Mirror image type, in which the aorta is interrupted distal to the ductus arteriosus, with a 98% chance of a congenital heart disease.

2. Right aortic arch with an aberrant left subclavian artery – this is due to interruption of the aortic development between the left subclavian and the left common carotid arteries. The aberrant subclavian artery is retrotracheal or retro-oesophageal. Association with congenital heart disease is low (5%).

Case 6.5

   A Crus of right hemidiaphragm

   B Gastric fundus

   C Spleen

   D Left sacroiliac joint

   E Right kidney

The crura of the diaphragm are fibrous bands that originate from the central tendon of the diaphragm and insert to either side of the upper lumbar vertebrae. They act as tethers for the muscular contraction of the diaphragm. The spleen has a marked variability of normal shape, particularly noticeable on CT, with small splenunculi again being a common CT finding.

Case 6.6

   A Right distal fibula

   B Base of right fifth metatarsal

   C Right navicular

   D Right Achilles tendon

   E Right cuboid

This question is rather simple provided the fundamental anatomy of the hind- and midfoot articulations is understood. The laterally positioned calcaneus articulates with the laterally placed cuboid, which in turn articulates with fourth and fifth metatarsals at the tarsometatarsal joint. The medially located talus articulates with the navicular, which in turn articulates with the medial, intermediate and lateral cuneiforms.

Case 6.7

   A Outer dural layer (periosteum)

   B Superior sagittal sinus

   C Subarachnoid space

   D Falx cerebri

   E Inner dural layer

The cerebral envelope consists of three layers and two spaces, as illustrated in **Figure 6.2**.

- **Extradural space** – a potential space between the skull vault and outer layer of the dura mater which is traversed by branches of meningeal arteries (a source of extradural haematoma)
- **Dura mater** – fibrous mater consisting of two layers, the outer and inner, which separate to enclose the dural venous sinuses

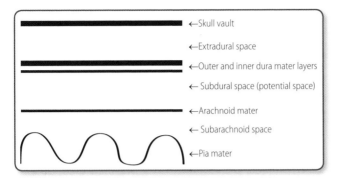

Figure 6.2 Schematic illustration of the cerebral envelope.

- **Subdural space** – potential space only, since dura and subarachnoid maters are closely applied together
- **Arachnoid mater** – avascular, lattice-like layer
- **Subarachnoid space** – contains cerebrospinal fluid
- **Pia mater** – vascular layer, closely applied to cerebral surface.

Case 6.8

A Right lesser trochanter

B Catheter balloon in navicular fossa

C Penile urethra

D Bulbous urethra

E Left hip joint

The male urethra has four anatomical parts, from proximal to distal: prostatic, membranous, bulbous and penile. To visualise the prostatic and membranous parts, the bladder is filled retrogradely with contrast before the patient is asked to void.

The navicular fossa is the most distal part of the penile urethra, in which the inflated catheter balloon can be seen in this example.

Case 6.9

A Sternocleidomastoid muscle

B Scalenus anterior muscle

C Subclavian artery

D Subclavian vein

E Clavicle

The subclavian vein and the phrenic nerve pass anterior to the scalenus anterior muscle whilst the subclavian artery and brachial plexus run posterior to it. Lesions in this region can involve the cords of the brachial plexus and cause neurological symptoms.

Case 6.10

A Right retromolar trigone

B Oropharynx

C Left masseter muscle

D Superficial lobe of the left parotid gland

E Cervical spinal cord

Axial anatomy of the neck is complex. It is useful to be familiar with anatomical landmarks to help with level orientation. Three main levels can be recognised: nasopharynx, oropharynx and hypopharynx.

The level of the oropharynx can be recognised by identifying the mandible and tongue.

The retromolar trigone is a triangular band of mucosa which lies posterior to the molar teeth at the level of the ramus of the mandible.

Case 6.11

A Left cephalic vein

B Left basilic vein

C Left median antecubital vein

D Left axillary vein

E Trochlea of the left humerus

Venous anatomy of the upper limb is highly variable. The cephalic vein runs on the radial aspect of the forearm and the outer aspect of the arm and usually drains into the axillary vein at the level of the shoulder joint. The basilic vein runs on the medial aspect of the arm. The brachial veins lie adjacent to the brachial artery and drain into the axillary vein.

The medial antecubital vein in the anterior aspect of the elbow is commonly used for intravenous cannulation.

Case 6.12

A Right anterior superior iliac spine

B Left semitendinosus muscle

C Right gracilis muscle

D Left adductor longus muscle

E Right femur

Sartorius is the longest muscle in the body that crosses two joints; the ipsilateral hip and knee joints. It originates from the anterior superior iliac spine (ASIS) and inserts into the pes anserine (proximal medial tibia).

An easy way to remember the origin of sartorius and rectus femoris is:

- ASIS – **S** for sartorius origin
- AIIS – rectus femoris muscle origin

To avoid confusing the proximal adductors and the quadriceps muscle groups, think of their relationships to the femur. The quadriceps muscles appear to 'hug' the femoral diaphysis, whereas the adductor group are seen in the medial thigh, away from the bone.

Case 6.13

A Head of epididymis

B Scrotal skin

C Tunica vaginalis

D Testis

E Aorta

Embryologically, the testes originate in the lumbar region before passing through the inguinal canal and eventually descending into the scrotum by the end of puberty. The blood supply relates to the site of origin of the testes, with each testis being supplied by a testicular artery which arises from the aorta just below the renal arteries. Each testicular vein forms from the pampiniform plexus of veins. The right testicular vein then drains to the inferior vena cava, whereas the left testicular vein drains to the left renal vein. For this reason, it is important to image the left kidney whenever a left-sided varicocoele is identified, as renal masses may cause this phenomenon. The lymphatic drainage of the testis is to the para-aortic nodes, which should be examined in the event of a testicular tumour being detected.

The tunica albuginea – the fibrous covering of the testis – is not usually seen on ultrasound unless a hydrocoele is present. The tunica vaginalis is a serous membrane which lies outwith the tunica albuginea and is seen as a hypoechoic ring around the testis on ultrasound.

Case 6.14

A Quadrigeminal cistern

B Cerebellar vermis

C Fourth ventricle

D Nodule of cerebellum

E Cisterna magna

With a bit of imagination the cerebellum and CSF spaces at this level resemble a face of a sad man with moustache (**Figure 6.3**): lateral ventricles form the eyes; quadrigeminal cistern – nose; fourth ventricle – mouth and cerebellar hemispheres – big moustache.

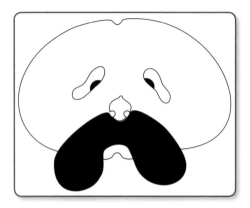

Figure 6.3 'Sad man with moustache' schematic illustration of the relationship between cerebellum and neighbouring CSF spaces in the coronal plane.

Case 6.15

  A Amnionic cavity

  B Vertebral column

  C Cerebrum

  D Nuchal thickness

  E Biparietal diameter

Measurements of nuchal thickness (the hypoechoic stripe in the posterior neck) are taken at 12 weeks' gestation, forming part of the estimation of risk of such anomalies as Down's syndrome. Usually this measurement is no more than 2 mm at this gestational age (up to 6 mm at 19 weeks' gestation). Whilst crown-rump length is used to estimate gestational age between 6.5 and 10 weeks' gestation, biparietal diameter is more accurate between 12 and 24 weeks. This is an axial measurement taken at the widest part of the calvarium, with the thalamus in the midline.

Case 6.16

  A Ossification centre of the right capitulum

  B Metaphysis of the base of the proximal phalanx of the little (fifth) finger

  C Ossification centre of the distal right radius

  D Right capitate

  E Ossification centre of the right thumb metacarpal

The presence of ossification centres on paediatric radiographs will allow an estimation of a child's age. Familiarise yourself with common milestones, most importantly the elbow.

Appearances of the ossification centres of the elbow = CRITOL, 1-3-5-7-9-11 is an easy way to remember the approximate dates of ossification:

C – Capitulum (1 year)

R – Radial head (3 years)

I – Medial (internal) epicondyle (5 years)

T – Trochlea (7 years)

O – Olecranon (9 years)

L – Lateral epicondyle (11 years.)

Case 6.17

A Conus medullaris

B Spinous process of L2

C Filum terminale

D Posterior longitudinal ligament

E Channel for basivertebral veins

The conus medullaris is the most inferior portion of the spinal cord, which in adults usually terminates at the L1–2 level. The filum terminale – a condensation of pia mater – continues inferiorly from the apex of the conus medullaris as a single fibrous strand which inserts into the posterior coccyx. A low-lying conus medullaris and thickening of the filum terminale (it should be less than 3 mm thick) are indicators of spinal dysraphism.

Case 6.18

A Right internal jugular vein

B Right true vocal cord

C Anterior commissure

D Left thyroid cartilage

E Left arytenoid cartilage

The vocal cords are situated within the larynx, protected by a cartilaginous skeleton which consists of the thyroid cartilage anteriorly, the signet-shaped cricoid cartilage posteriorly and the epiglottis superiorly. The anterior margins of the true vocal cords are connected by the anterior commissure and the posterior margins are attached to the arytenoid cartilages.

The false (vestibular) vocal cords are a pair of thick folds of mucosa which lie superior to the true vocal cords. To distinguish them from the true vocal cords, one should look for the arytenoids cartilages – if not seen posteriorly, one is looking at the false cords.

Case 6.19

A Right bronchial artery

B Right first intercostal artery

C Anterior spinal artery

D Right atrium

E Three

Bronchial arterial anatomy is variable. Usually, there is a single artery on the right and two on the left, all arising from the aorta. In chronic pulmonary conditions such as cystic fibrosis, these arteries can enlarge, become friable and, as their blood pressure reaches systemic levels, can lead to haemoptysis which may require embolisation.

The anterior spinal arteries may arise from the bronchial arteries and it is important to ensure that these are not inadvertently embolised as this may lead to spinal cord damage and paralysis.

Case 6.20

A Femur

B Vastus intermedius muscle

C Gracilis muscle

D Long head of biceps femoris muscle

E Sartorius muscle

The muscles of the thigh are divided into the anterior, medial and posterior compartments. The muscles within each compartment are as follows:

Anterior compartment

- Tensor fascia lata
- Quadriceps muscles (rectus femoris, vastus medialis, vastus intermedius and vastus lateralis)
- Sartorius

Medial compartment

- Gracilis
- Adductor muscles (adductor brevis, adductor longus and adductor magnus)

Posterior compartment

- Hamstring muscles (long head of biceps femoris, semimembranosus and semitendinosus)
- Short head of biceps femoris

Remember, the anatomical compartmental division of the thigh muscles differs from the functional groupings.

Chapter 7

Mock paper 7

20 cases to be answered in 75 minutes

Case 7.1

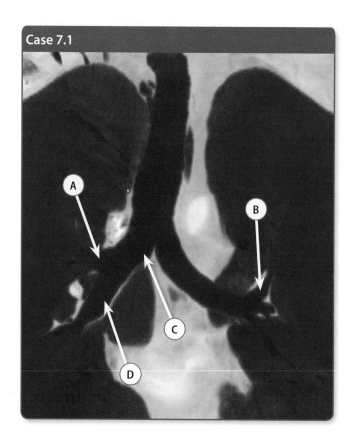

Case 7.1

QUESTION		WRITE YOUR ANSWER HERE
A	Name the structure labelled A.	
B	Name the structure labelled B.	
C	Name the structure labelled C.	
D	Name the structure labelled D.	
E	What is the normal total number of bronchopulmonary segments?	

Case 7.2

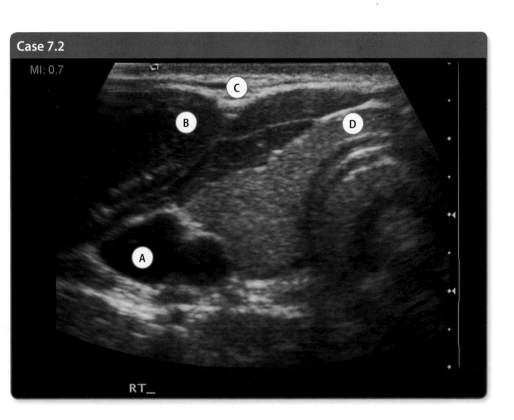

	MI: 0.7

RT_

Case 7.2

QUESTION		WRITE YOUR ANSWER HERE
A	Name the structure labelled A.	
B	Name the structure labelled B.	
C	Name the fibrous structure labelled C.	
D	Name the structure labelled D.	
E	Which nerve runs in the carotid sheath?	

Case 7.3

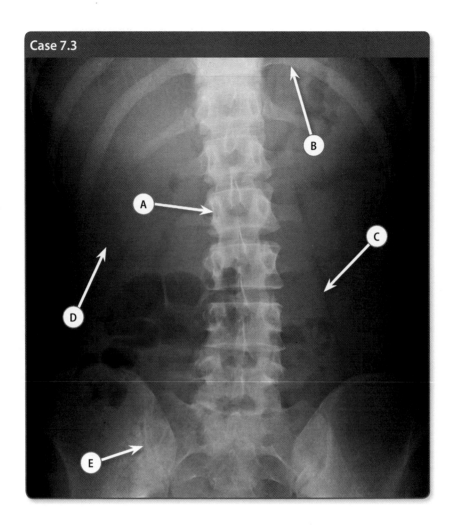

Case 7.3

QUESTION		WRITE YOUR ANSWER HERE
A	Name the structure labelled A.	
B	Name the structure labelled B.	
C	Name the structure labelled C.	
D	Name the structure labelled D.	
E	Name the structure labelled E.	

Case 7.4

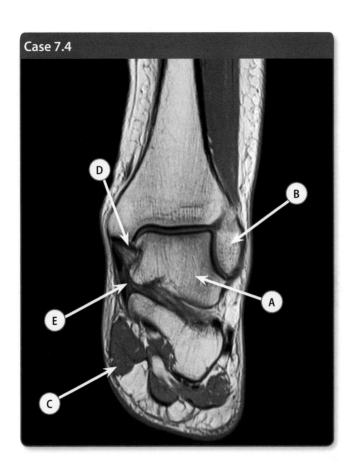

Case 7.4

QUESTION		WRITE YOUR ANSWER HERE
A	Name the structure labelled A.	
B	Name the structure labelled B.	
C	Name the structure labelled C.	
D	Name the structure labelled D.	
E	Name the structure labelled E.	

Case 7.5

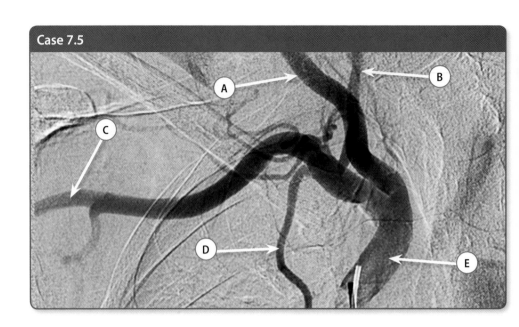

Case 7.5

QUESTION		WRITE YOUR ANSWER HERE
A	Name the structure labelled A.	
B	Name the structure labelled B.	
C	Name the structure labelled C.	
D	Name the structure labelled D.	
E	Name the structure labelled E.	

Case 7.6

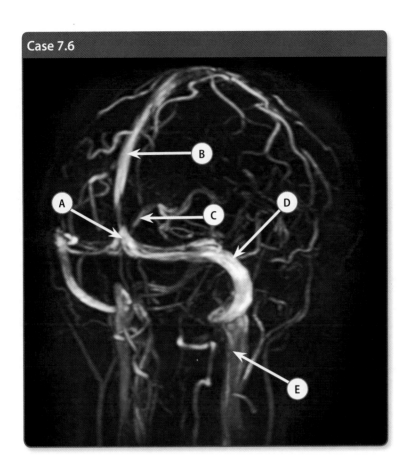

Case 7.6	
QUESTION	**WRITE YOUR ANSWER HERE**
A	Name the structure labelled A.	
B	Name the structure labelled B.	
C	Name the structure labelled C.	
D	Name the structure labelled D.	
E	Name the structure labelled E.	

Case 7.7

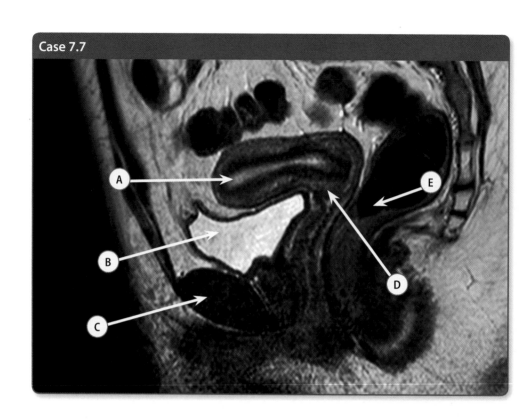

Case 7.7

QUESTION		WRITE YOUR ANSWER HERE
A	Name the structure labelled A.	
B	Name the structure labelled B.	
C	Name the structure labelled C.	
D	Name the structure labelled D.	
E	Name the structure labelled E.	

Case 7.8

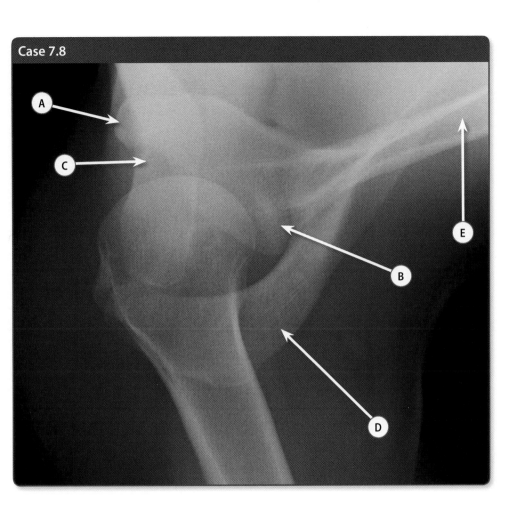

Case 7.8

QUESTION		WRITE YOUR ANSWER HERE
A	Name the structure labelled A.	
B	Name the structure labelled B.	
C	Name the structure labelled C.	
D	Name the structure labelled D.	
E	Name the structure labelled E.	

Case 7.9

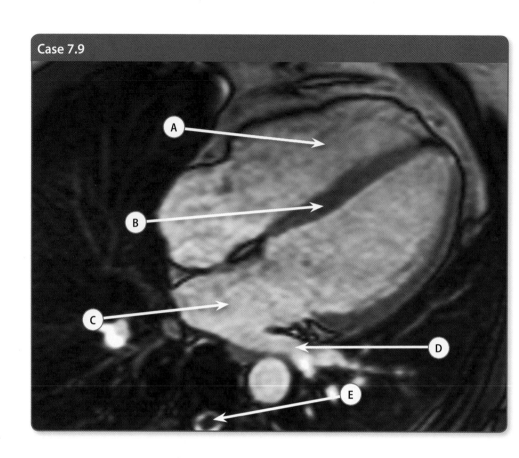

Case 7.9

QUESTION		WRITE YOUR ANSWER HERE
A	Name the chamber labelled A.	
B	Name the structure labelled B.	
C	Name the chamber labelled C.	
D	Name the structure labelled D.	
E	Name the structure labelled E.	

Case 7.10

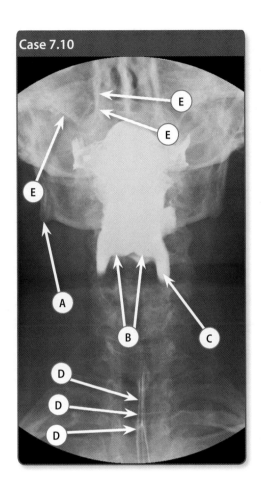

	QUESTION	WRITE YOUR ANSWER HERE
A	Name the structure labelled A.	
B	What structure is causing the impression labelled B?	
C	Name the structure labelled C.	
D	Name the structure labelled D.	
E	Name the structure labelled E.	

Case 7.11

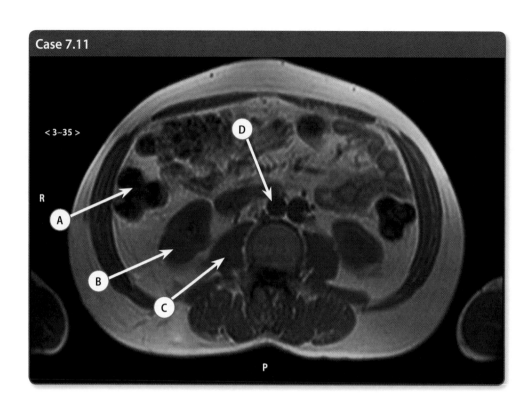

< 3–35 >

Case 7.11

QUESTION		WRITE YOUR ANSWER HERE
A	Name the structure labelled A.	
B	Name the structure labelled B.	
C	Name the structure labelled C.	
D	Name the arterial structure labelled D.	
E	Which anatomical variant is present on this image?	

Case 7.12

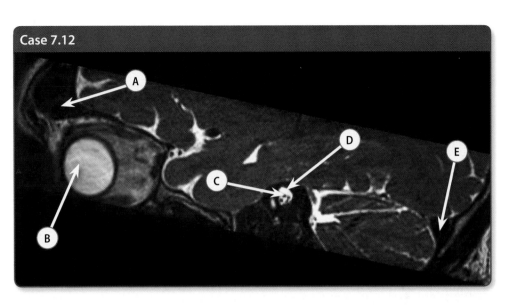

Case 7.12

QUESTION		WRITE YOUR ANSWER HERE
A	Name the structure labelled A.	
B	Name the structure labelled B.	
C	Name the structure labelled C.	
D	Name the structure labelled D.	
E	Name the structure labelled E.	

Case 7.13

RIGHT

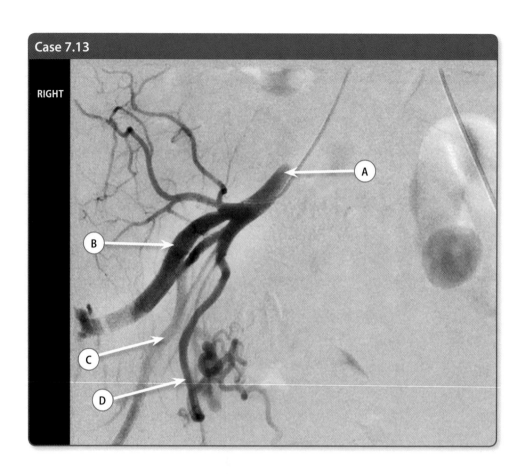

Case 7.13

QUESTION		WRITE YOUR ANSWER HERE
A	Name the structure labelled A.	
B	Name the structure labelled B.	
C	Name the structure labelled C.	
D	Name the structure labelled D.	
E	Name one branch of the posterior trunk of the internal iliac artery.	

Case 7.14

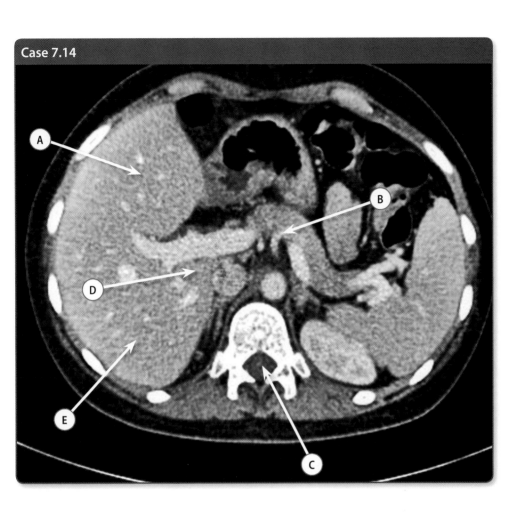

Case 7.14

QUESTION		WRITE YOUR ANSWER HERE
A	Name the liver segment labelled A.	
B	Name the structure labelled B.	
C	Name the structure labelled C.	
D	Name the liver segment labelled D.	
E	Name the liver segment labelled E.	

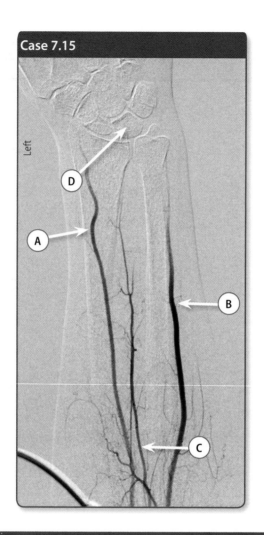

Case 7.15

Left

D

A

B

C

Case 7.15		
QUESTION		**WRITE YOUR ANSWER HERE**
A	Name the structure labelled A.	
B	Name the structure labelled B.	
C	Name the structure labelled C.	
D	Name the structure labelled D.	
E	What artery divides into two major branches A and B at the level of the elbow?	

Case 7.16

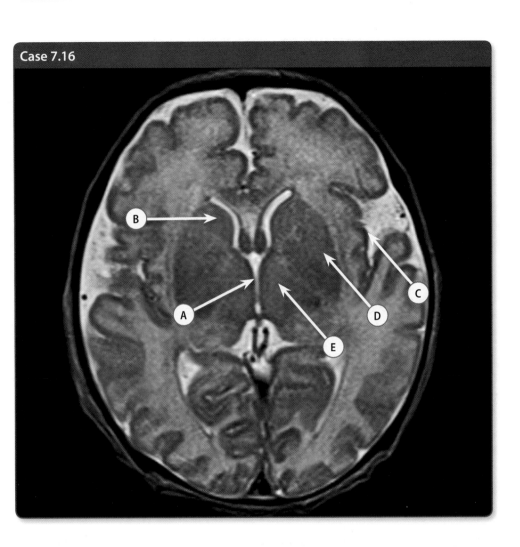

Case 7.16

QUESTION		WRITE YOUR ANSWER HERE
A	Name the structure labelled A.	
B	Name the structure labelled B.	
C	Name the structure labelled C.	
D	Name the structure labelled D.	
E	Name the structure labelled E.	

Case 7.17

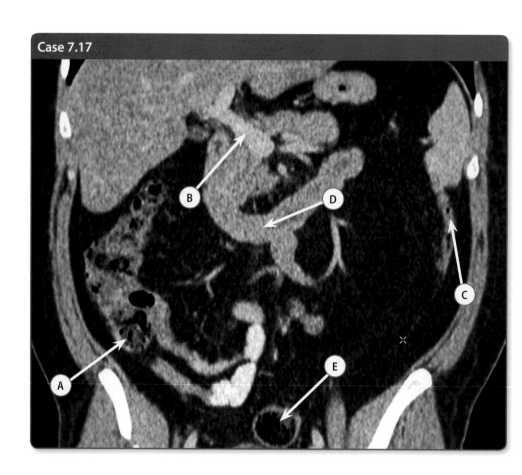

Case 7.17

QUESTION		WRITE YOUR ANSWER HERE
A	Name the structure labelled A.	
B	Name the structure labelled B.	
C	Name the structure labelled C.	
D	Name the structure labelled D.	
E	Name the structure labelled E.	

Case 7.18

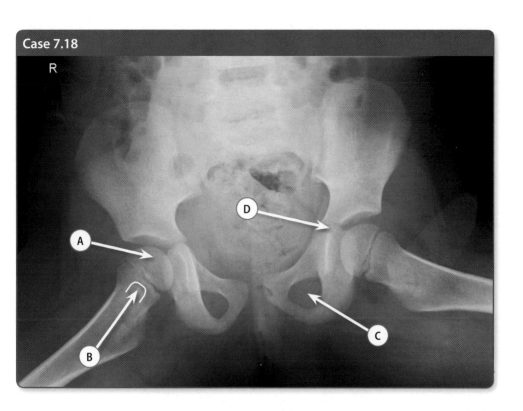

Case 7.18

QUESTION		WRITE YOUR ANSWER HERE
A	Name the structure labelled A.	
B	Name the structure labelled B.	
C	Name the structure labelled C.	
D	Name the structure labelled D.	
E	What is the name given to this radiographic view?	

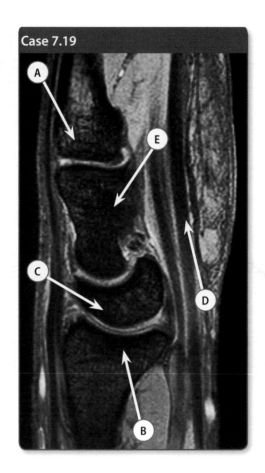

Case 7.19

Case 7.19		
QUESTION		**WRITE YOUR ANSWER HERE**
A	Name the structure labelled A.	
B	Name the structure labelled B.	
C	Name the structure labelled C.	
D	Name the structure labelled D.	
E	Name the structure labelled E.	

Case 7.20

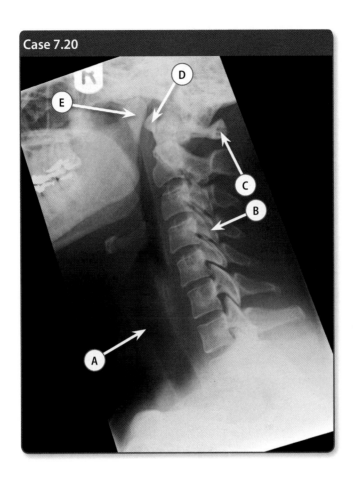

Case 7.20

QUESTION		WRITE YOUR ANSWER HERE
A	Name the structure labelled A.	
B	Name the structure labelled B.	
C	Name the structure labelled C.	
D	Name the structure labelled D.	
E	Name the structure labelled E.	

Answers

Case 7.1

A Right upper lobe bronchus

B Left upper lobe bronchus

C Right main bronchus

D Bronchus intermedius

E 18

Each bronchopulmonary segment is supplied by a segmental bronchus of the same name. A summary is given in **Table 7.1**.

Table 7.1 Segmental architecture of the lungs

Right lung	Left lung
Upper lobe	
Apical segment	Apicoposterior segment
Posterior segment	
Anterior segment	
Middle lobe	**Lingula (upper lobe)**
Lateral segment	Superior lingular segment
Medial segment	Inferior lingular segment
Lower lobe	
Superior (apical) segment	
Anterior basal segment	Anteromedial basal segment
Medial basal segment	
Lateral basal segment	
Posterior basal segment	

Case 7.2

A Right internal jugular vein

B Right sternocleidomastoid muscle

C Deep cervical fascia

D Thyroid isthmus

E Vagus nerve (X)

This US image shows structures in the neck at level VI and you should be able to orientate yourself by the:

- Thyroid isthmus, located inferior to the cricoid cartilage and medial to the sternocleidomastoid muscle
- Common carotid artery which divides to internal and external branches above the superior margin of the thyroid cartilage.

Case 7.3

A Right pedicle of L2

B Left 11th rib

C Left psoas major outline

D Right lobe of liver

E Right sacroiliac joint

Normal amounts of gas are present in the stomach and scattered throughout the large bowel. There is normally minimal or no gas in the small bowel lumen. The more intra-abdominal fat a patient has, the the more readily visible the outlines of the normal viscera and muscles. This body habitus is also beneficial when viewing CT images as the low attenuation fat makes the organs stand out. The worst patients for abdominal CT and plain films are the very thin! This is a complete contrast to ultrasound, in which the ideal patient would be as thin as possible.

Case 7.4

A Talus

B Lateral malleolus

C Abductor hallucis muscle

D Deltoid ligament – deep band

E Deltoid ligament – superficial band

The deltoid ligament (medial collateral ligamentous complex) is found deep to the medial flexor tendons (tibialis posterior, flexor digitorum longus and flexor hallucis longus tendons – remember the mnemonic 'Tom, Dick and Harry'). It has several components, although the tibiotalar and tibiocalcaneal fibres are only routinely visualised on coronal MR. These are termed the deep and superficial bands respectively. The deep tibiotalar portion courses diagonally between the medial malleolus and the talus. The superficial tibiocalcaneal band runs more vertically, deep to the flexor retinaculum and superficial to the tibiotalar component of the ligament.

Case 7.5

   A Right common carotid artery

   B Right vertebral artery

   C Right axillary artery

   D Right internal thoracic/mammary artery

   E Brachiocephalic trunk/innominate artery

A mnemonic to remember the branches of the subclavian artery is **VIT C: V**ertebral, **I**nternal thoracic, **T**hyrocervical trunk, **C**ostocervical trunk.

There are no branches of the vertebral artery in the neck. The internal thoracic artery terminates by dividing into the superior epigastric and the superior phrenic arteries. The thyrocervical trunk divides into three branches – the **S**uprascapular, **I**nferior thyroid and **T**ransverse cervical arteries (**SIT**). The costocervical trunk divides into the deep cervical and the highest intercostal arteries.

From the outer aspect of the first rib, the subclavian artery continues as the axillary artery.

Case 7.6

   A Confluence of the venous sinuses (torcular herophili)

   B Superior sagittal sinus

   C Straight sinus

   D Right transverse sinus

   E Right internal jugular vein

Blood from the deep cerebral veins drains centrally into the dural sinuses (the vascular channels lying between the layers of dura). The superior sagittal, straight and occipital sinuses meet at the venous confluence, also known as the torcular herophili. The venous confluence divides into two transverse sinuses which drain into the internal jugular veins via the sigmoid sinuses.

Case 7.7

   A Endometrial cavity

   B Bladder

   C Symphysis pubis

   D Cervix

   E Rectum

The uterus in this example is anteverted and anteflexed and demonstrates the characteristic trilaminar appearance of the endometrium. Note the relationship of the cervix which lies anterior to the rectum.

Sagittal views through the pelvis might show numerous important anatomical structures and their relationship to other pelvic organs. Candidates must be able to recognise all the major structures confidently and not just the organs relating to an individual anatomical system. Vertebral bodies, discs and nerve roots may also be visible and candidates are expected to recognise and name them.

Case 7.8

A Coracoid process

B Glenoid of scapula

C Clavicle (lateral part)

D Acromion

E Body of scapula

Osseous anatomy of the shoulder is fundamental knowledge for the examination. Several radiographic projections of the shoulder may be acquired (this is an axial view) – the following are a few tips to help orientate you if presented with an unusual projection:

1. The coracoid process always 'points' anteriorly
2. The acromion articulates with the clavicle at the acromioclavicular joint
3. The head of humerus articulates with the glenoid of scapula at the glenohumeral joint

Remember, the coracoid process does not articulate with an osseous structure distally. This will allow you to easily differentiate between the coracoid and acromion.

Case 7.9

A Right ventricle

B Interventricular septum (muscular part)

C Left atrium

D Left inferior pulmonary vein

E Spinal cord

On axial imaging, the right ventricle is the most anterior chamber of the heart with the left atrium being the most posterior chamber. The right atrium is posterolateral to the right ventricle and to the right of it. The left ventricle lies posterolateral and to the left of the right ventricle. These relationships can be appreciated in **Figure 7.1**.

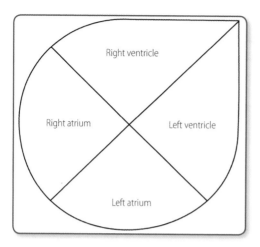

Figure 7.1 The relative positions of the cardiac chambers on an axial view.

Case 7.10

A Angle of right mandible

B Epiglottis

C Left piriform recess

D Oesophagus

E Right maxillary sinus

The pharynx consists of three parts (from superior to inferior): nasopharynx; oropharynx; and laryngopharynx (hypopharynx). The latter two parts are shown filled with barium in this image. The laryngopharynx extends from the tip of the epiglottis to the point at which the pharynx becomes the oesophagus (at the level of the C6 vertebra). The piriform recesses are parts of the laryngopharynx and pass laterally to the larynx.

Case 7.11

A Ascending colon

B Right kidney

C Right psoas muscle

D Aorta

E Left-sided inferior vena cava

This is a T1-weighted axial sequence at the level of L2, in which the inferior vena cava (IVC) lies to the left of the aorta. This is a variation of normal and is a congenital variant. Several types exist but typically the left IVC terminates at the left renal vein and then crosses at the usual position to the right of the aorta. The IVC usually has a larger diameter than the aorta, a useful hint when trying to accurately label and identify the central vasculature on a single cross-sectional slice.

Case 7.12

  A Frontal sinus

  B Globe

  C Facial nerve (VII)

  D Internal acoustic meatus

  E Transverse venous sinus

The facial nerve (VII) and three divisions of the vestibulocochlear nerve (VII) – cochlear nerve, superior vestibular branch and inferior vestibular branch – pass through the internal acoustic meatus (IAM). **Figure 7.2** depicts their relative positions in the IAM.

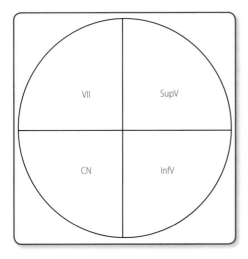

Figure 7.2 Relative positions of VII and VIII branches in the internal acoustic meatus. SupV, superior vestibular branch of vestibulocochlear nerve (VIII); CN, cochlear nerve; InfV, inferior vestibular branch VIII; VII, facial nerve.

Here, the mnemonic comes useful to remember their relative position: 'Seven up, Coke down'

Seven **up** – Seventh (VII) nerve is located **superiorly** and **anteriorly**

Coke **down** – The Cochlear nerve is located **inferiorly** and **anteriorly.**

Case 7.13

  A Right common iliac artery

  B Right external iliac artery

  C Posterior trunk of internal iliac artery

  D Right uterine artery

  E Iliolumbar/lateral sacral/superior gluteal artery

The internal iliac artery has anterior and posterior trunks. The uterine artery most commonly arises from the anterior trunk and takes a horizontal route to supply the uterus. The posterior division gives off the iliolumbar, lateral sacral and superior gluteal branches.

The posterior branches can be easily remembered with the mnemonic **PILS: P**osterior: **I**liolumbar, **L**ateral sacral, **S**uperior gluteal.

Case 7.14

A Segment IVb

B Splenic artery

C Spinal cord

D Segment I (caudate lobe)

E Segment VI

The Couinaud classification divides the liver anatomy into eight segments, all with independent function. Each segment is centred on branches of the portal vein, hepatic artery and bile duct. In the periphery of each segment vascular outflow is provided via the hepatic veins.

Segment I is anatomically different from the other segments. It drains directly in the IVC. Note that the caudate lobe lies between the portal vein and the IVC.

Case 7.15

A Left radial artery

B Left ulnar artery

C Left interosseous artery

D Left lunate

E Left brachial artery

The brachial artery is the major arterial supply of the arm. This begins at the lower border of the teres major muscle and usually divides at the elbow into the radial and ulnar arteries. This bifurcation is highly variable and sometimes occurs in the upper arm.

The branches of the brachial artery are the profunda brachii, superior and inferior ulnar collateral arteries, nutrient artery to humerus and its terminal branches.

The interosseous artery is a branch of the ulnar artery and divides into anterior and posterior divisions.

Case 7.16

A Third ventricle

B Head of the right caudate nucleus

C Cortex of the left insula

D Left lentiform nucleus

E Left hypothalamus

The MRI appearances of the neonatal brain differ significantly from that of an adult. As the myelination process has not fully completed at birth, the neonatal brain is 'wetter' than the adult brain, resulting in reversed T1 and T2 signal characteristics (i.e. white matter returns low signal on T1- and high on T2-weighted MRI).

At birth, only the myelinated posterior fossa structures (such as the brainstem, cerebellum and the posterior limb of the internal capsule) have adult appearances. It is important to recognise that these differences relate to normal anatomy and are not pathological.

Case 7.17

A Caecum

B Portal vein

C Descending colon

D Third part of the duodenum

E Gas in sigmoid colon

The portal vein is responsible for draining the blood from the gastrointestinal system into the liver. It is formed by the confluence of the superior mesenteric and splenic veins, behind the neck of the pancreas. At the porta hepatis it branches into right and left intrahepatic portal veins to supply the corresponding hepatic lobes.

Case 7.18

A Right capital femoral epiphysis

B Right greater trochanter

C Left obturator foramen

D Triradiate cartilage of the left acetabulum

E 'Frog leg'

This is a 'frog leg' pelvic radiograph which is performed with the patient's knees flexed and the thighs maximally abducted. The primary purpose of this view is to assess for the presence of slipped capital femoral epiphyses, which are usually rendered more conspicuous than on a standard AP view with posteromedial displacement of the femoral head. On the frog leg lateral view, the greater trochanter is visualised en face, projected through the proximal femur. The Y-shaped triradiate cartilage is the point at which the ilium, ischium and pubis meet; this usually fuses by 20 years of age.

Case 7.19

  A Base of third metacarpal

  B Distal radius

  C Lunate

  D Flexor digitorum superficialis tendon

  E Capitate

This selected sagittal MRI of the wrist demonstrates the straight alignment of the distal radius, lunate, capitate and base of the third metacarpal. If this alignment is disrupted, one must consider a lunate or perilunate dislocation has occurred.

TIP: there is more soft tissue 'padding' on the palmar aspect of the hand in comparison with the dorsal aspect. When trying to determine if an extensor or flexor tendon is labelled, remember that flexors will be on the 'thicker' side of the hand, i.e. the palmar aspect.

Case 7.20

  A Trachea

  B Inferior articular process of C4

  C Posterior tubercle of C1

  D Anterior arch of C1

  E Right mandibular condyle

An adequate lateral cervical spine radiograph will visualise the C7/T1 junction (as in this case). The inferior and superior articular processes articulate at the facet joints, which slope posteroinferiorly and should overlap (or lie closely parallel) in a normal, non-rotated radiograph.

Chapter 8

Mock paper 8

20 cases to be answered in 75 minutes

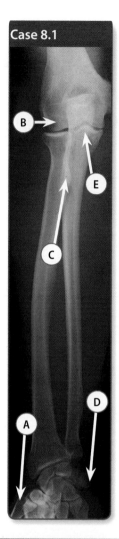

Case 8.1

	QUESTION	WRITE YOUR ANSWER HERE
A	Name the structure labelled A.	
B	Name the structure labelled B.	
C	Name the tendon that attaches to the structure labelled C.	
D	Name the structure labelled D.	
E	Name the structure labelled E.	

Case 8.2

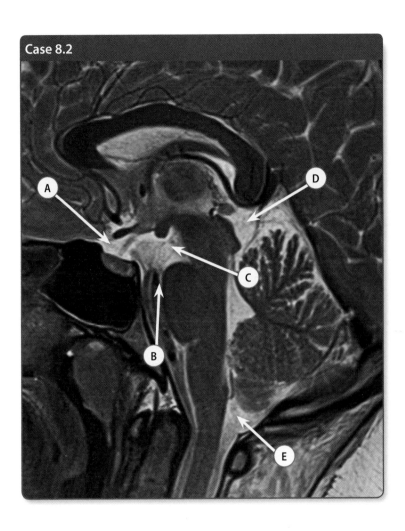

Case 8.2

QUESTION		WRITE YOUR ANSWER HERE
A	Name the space labelled A.	
B	Name the space labelled B.	
C	Name the space labelled C.	
D	Name the space labelled D.	
E	Name the space labelled E.	

Case 8.3

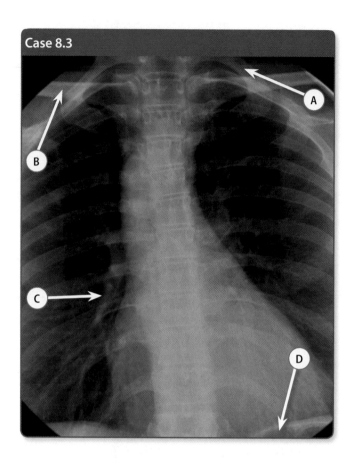

Case 8.3

QUESTION		WRITE YOUR ANSWER HERE
A	Name the structure labelled A.	
B	Name the structure labelled B.	
C	Name the structure labelled C.	
D	In which structure does the gas labelled D lie?	
E	Which anatomical variant is present on this image?	

Case 8.4

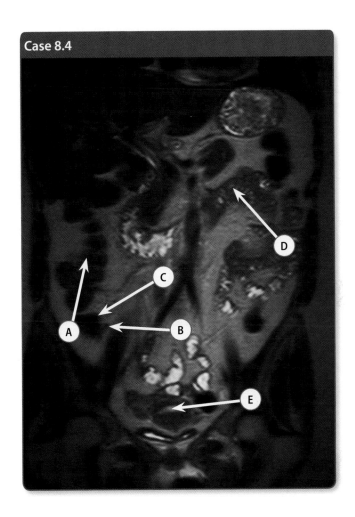

Case 8.4	
QUESTION	**WRITE YOUR ANSWER HERE**
A Name the structure labelled A.	
B Name the structure labelled B.	
C Name the structure labelled C.	
D Name the structure labelled D.	
E Name the structure labelled E.	

Case 8.5

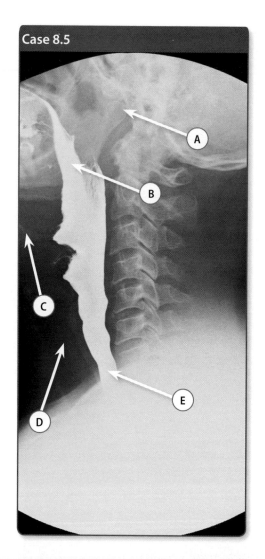

Case 8.5

QUESTION		WRITE YOUR ANSWER HERE
A	Name the structure labelled A.	
B	Name the structure labelled B.	
C	Name the structure labelled C.	
D	Name the lucent structure labelled D.	
E	Name the structure labelled E.	

Case 8.6

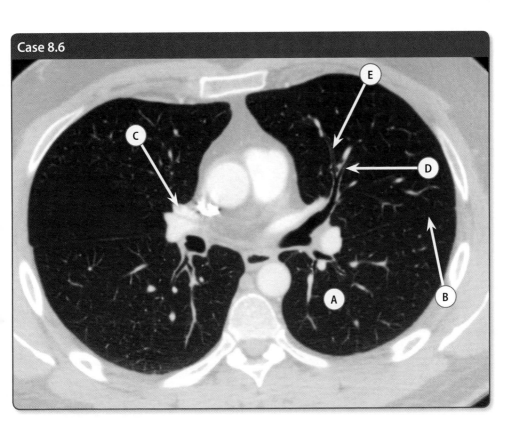

Case 8.6

QUESTION		WRITE YOUR ANSWER HERE
A	What lung lobe is labelled A?	
B	Name the structure labelled B.	
C	Name the structure labelled C.	
D	Name the structure labelled D.	
E	Name the structure labelled E.	

Case 8.7

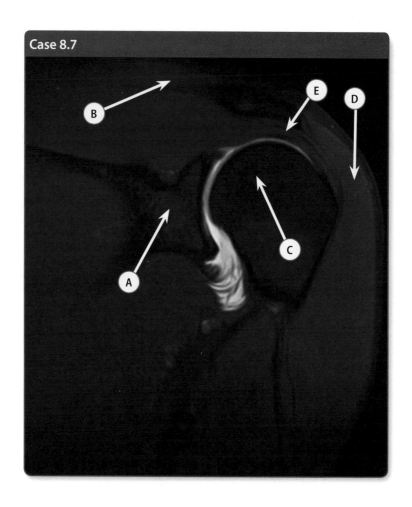

Case 8.7

QUESTION		WRITE YOUR ANSWER HERE
A	Name the structure labelled A.	
B	Name the structure labelled B.	
C	Name the structure labelled C.	
D	Name the structure labelled D.	
E	Name the structure labelled E.	

Case 8.8

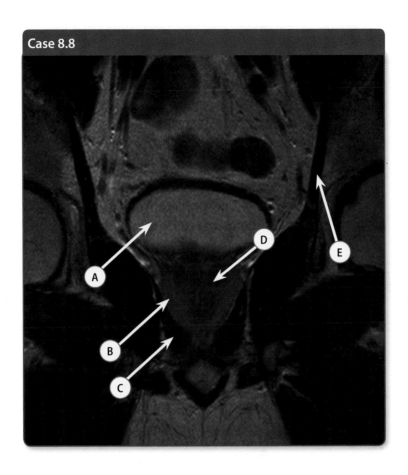

Case 8.8

QUESTION		WRITE YOUR ANSWER HERE
A	Name the structure labelled A.	
B	Name the structure labelled B.	
C	Name the structure labelled C.	
D	Name the structure labelled D.	
E	Name the structure labelled E.	

Case 8.9

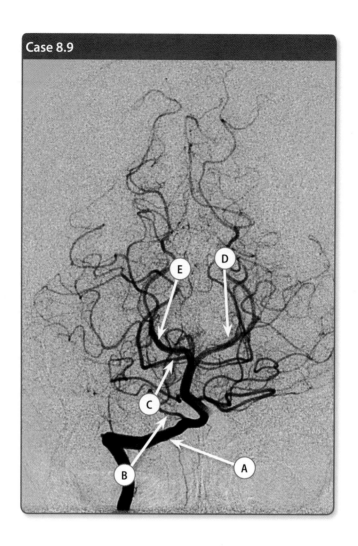

Case 8.9

QUESTION		WRITE YOUR ANSWER HERE
A	Name the structure labelled A.	
B	Name the structure labelled B.	
C	Name the structure labelled C.	
D	Name the structure labelled D.	
E	Name the structure labelled E.	

Case 8.10

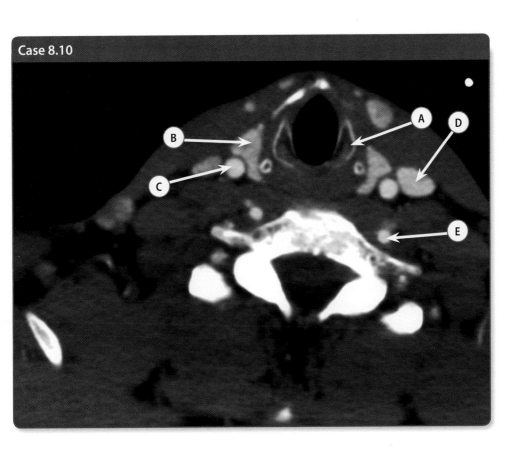

Case 8.10

QUESTION	WRITE YOUR ANSWER HERE
A Name the structure labelled A.	
B Name the structure labelled B.	
C Name the structure labelled C.	
D Name the structure labelled D.	
E Name the structure labelled E.	

Case 8.11

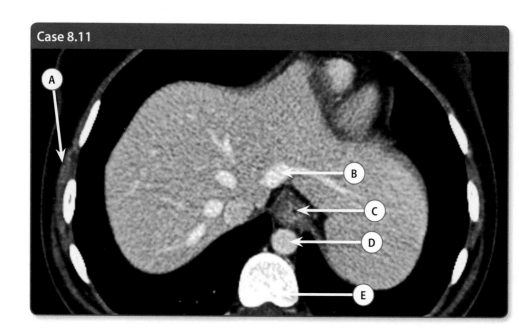

Case 8.11

QUESTION		WRITE YOUR ANSWER HERE
A	Name the structure labelled A.	
B	Name the structure labelled B.	
C	Name the structure labelled C.	
D	Name the structure labelled D.	
E	Name the structure labelled E.	

Case 8.12

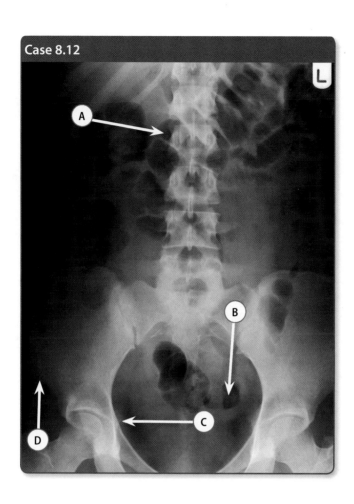

	QUESTION	WRITE YOUR ANSWER HERE
A	What part of the colon is labelled A?	
B	What part of the colon is labelled B?	
C	Name the bony prominence labelled C.	
D	Name the structure labelled D.	
E	What muscle exits the pelvis through the greater sciatic foramen?	

Case 8.13

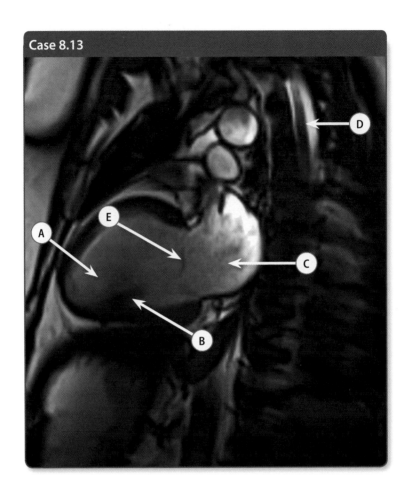

Case 8.13

QUESTION		WRITE YOUR ANSWER HERE
A	Name the chamber labelled A.	
B	Name the structure labelled B.	
C	Name the chamber labelled C.	
D	Name the structure labelled D.	
E	Name the structure labelled E.	

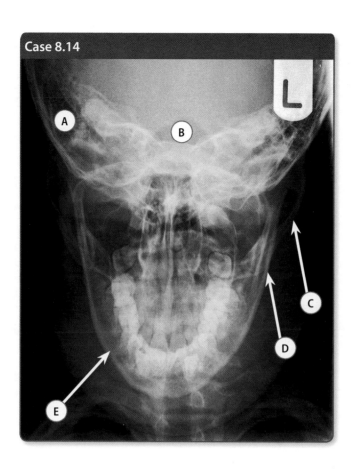

Case 8.14

QUESTION	WRITE YOUR ANSWER HERE
A	Name the structure labelled A.	
B	Name the structure labelled B.	
C	Name the structure labelled C.	
D	Name the structure labelled D.	
E	Name the structure labelled E.	

Case 8.15

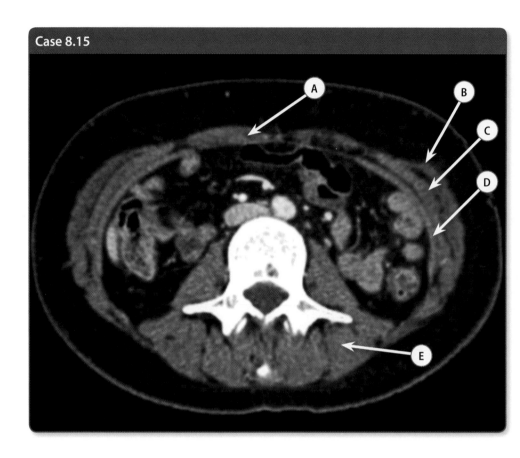

Case 8.15

QUESTION		WRITE YOUR ANSWER HERE
A	Name the structure labelled A.	
B	Name the structure labelled B.	
C	Name the structure labelled C.	
D	Name the structure labelled D.	
E	Name the structure labelled E.	

Case 8.16

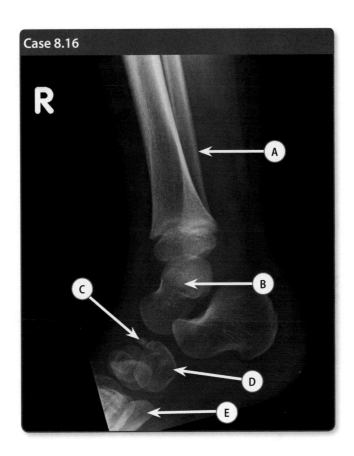

Case 8.16

QUESTION		WRITE YOUR ANSWER HERE
A	Name the structure labelled A.	
B	Name the structure labelled B.	
C	Name the structure labelled C.	
D	Name the structure labelled D.	
E	Name the structure labelled E.	

Case 8.17

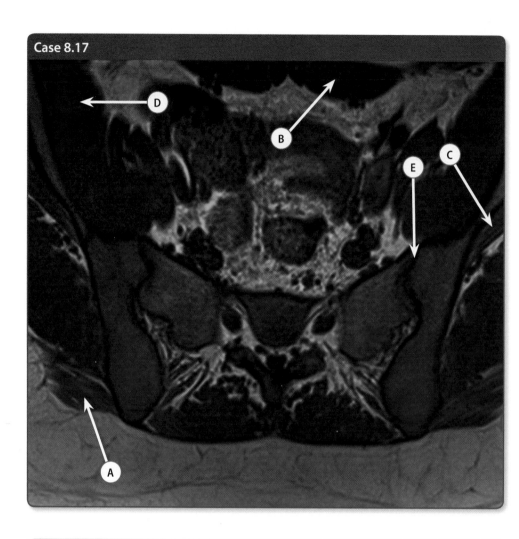

Case 8.17

QUESTION		WRITE YOUR ANSWER HERE
A	Name the structure labelled A.	
B	Name the structure labelled B.	
C	Name the insertion site of the structure labelled C.	
D	Name the structure labelled D.	
E	Name the structure labelled E.	

Case 8.18

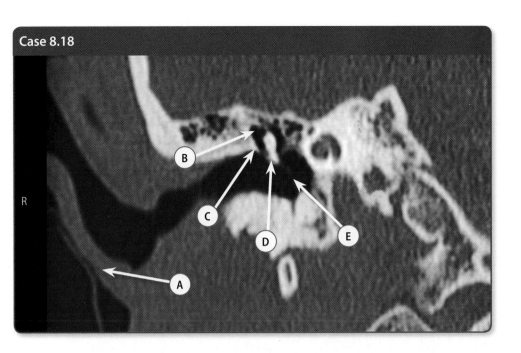

Case 8.18 Axial CT at the level of C5

QUESTION	WRITE YOUR ANSWER HERE
A Name the structure labelled A.	
B Name the structure labelled B.	
C Name the structure labelled C.	
D Name the structure labelled D.	
E Name the structure labelled E.	

Case 8.19

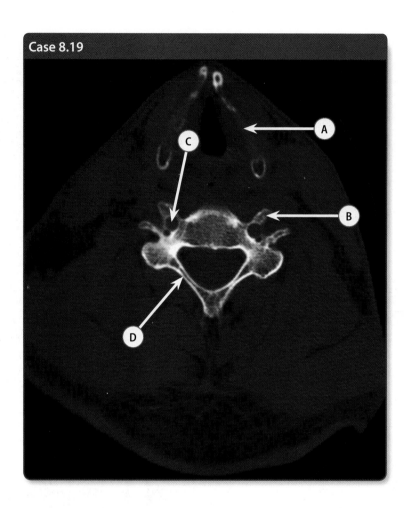

Case 8.19 Axial CT at the level of C5

QUESTION		WRITE YOUR ANSWER HERE
A	Name the structure labelled A.	
B	Name the structure labelled B.	
C	What structure passes through the structure labelled C?	
D	Name the structure labelled D.	
E	Which anatomical variant is present on this image?	

Case 8.20

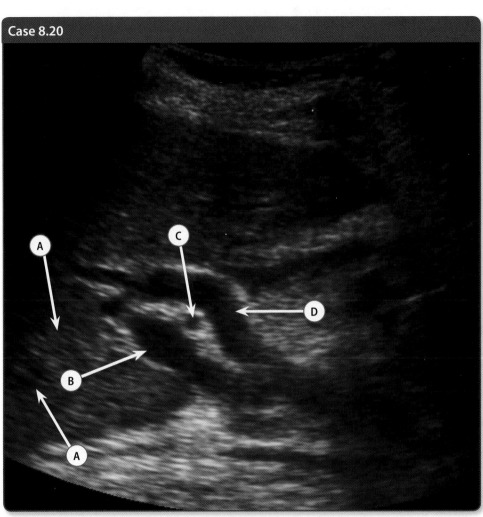

Case 8.20

QUESTION		WRITE YOUR ANSWER HERE
A	Name the structure labelled A.	
B	Name the structure labelled B.	
C	Name the structure labelled C.	
D	Name the structure labelled D.	
E	In what direction does portal venous flow relative to the liver?	

Answers

Case 8.1

A Base of the metacarpal of the thumb

B Capitulum of humerus

C Biceps brachii muscle

D Pisiform

E Coronoid process of ulna

There is lots of osseous anatomy on this single radiograph and the following step-by-step technique should be utilised during the examination as a fail-safe measure to answer everything correctly:

- It is clear that (A) is the base of a metacarpal but knowing the following point will allow you to confidently answer that it is the metacarpal of the thumb:
  - it is seen on the radial aspect of radiograph
  - the radius is laterally positioned

- the distal humerus articulates with both the radius and ulna
  - the capitulum (B) articulates with the head of radius
  - the trochlea articulates with the proximal ulna

- the sesamoid pisiform bone (D) is located on the ulnar aspect of the proximal carpal row and only articulates with the triquetral

- the coronoid process of the ulna (E) is shown as a triangular projection filling the groove within the trochlea of the distal humerus.

Case 8.2

A Suprasellar cistern

B Prepontine cistern

C Interpeduncular cistern

D Quadrigeminal cistern

E Cisterna magna

The arachnoid and pia matter are applied closely together but become separate at the base of the brain and around the brainstem to form a system of subarachnoid cisterns. The cisterns are usually named after their relationships with adjacent structures, such as the prepontine cistern (pons), suprasellar cistern (sella turcica) or cisterna magna (foramen magnum). The cisterns communicate with each other, thus allowing free flow of CSF between them. Some of the cerebral arteries and cranial nerves course within the cisterns.

Case 8.3

A Left first rib

B Right clavicle

C Right lower lobe pulmonary artery

D Gastric fundus

E Right aortic arch

The asymptomatic adult variant of a right aortic arch is usually associated with an aberrant left subclavian artery. This can cause a posterior indentation of the oesophagus on a barium swallow.

This can be identified on a chest radiograph using the following clues:

1. Ensure the radiograph is appropriately orientated (side marker)
2. Appreciate the lack of a left sided arch above the left pulmonary artery
3. Ensure that the heart is normally sited, i.e. there is no dextrocardia.

Case 8.4

A Ascending colon

B Appendix

C Ileocaecal valve/caecum

D Duodenojejunal junction

E Endometrial cavity of the uterus

Many authorities have now stated that when reviewing and reporting abdominal and pelvic CT or MRI, it is essential to include coronal assessment. Reliance on axial imaging is no longer acceptable as the extra information gained from coronal and, where necessary, sagittal imaging, is significant in many cases. The inclusion of coronal and sagittal body imaging will become more commonplace in radiological examinations, so ensure you know your way around these types of images.

This particular MRI shows the value of coronal imaging in demonstrating the peritoneal spaces, recesses and reflections.

Case 8.5

A Mandibular condyle

B Oropharynx

C Hyoid bone

D Trachea

E Oesophagus

The oesophagus is a continuation of the oropharynx. Beginning at the level of C6, it descends posteriorly to the trachea, just anterior to the lower cervical vertebrae (hence osteophytic compression is a not uncommon cause of dysphagia).

Case 8.6

A Left lower lobe

B Left oblique fissure

C Right superior pulmonary vein

D Inferior lingular segment bronchus

E Superior lingular segment bronchus

The lingula of the left lung is homologous to the middle lobe of the right lung. The lingula is composed of the superior and inferior lingular segments. Being adjacent to the left heart border, consolidation in the lingula will result in loss of the left heart border silhouette, an important radiographic finding.

Case 8.7

A Glenoid of shoulder

B Trapezius muscle

C Head of humerus

D Deltoid muscle

E Supraspinatus muscle (musculotendinous portion)

MRI of the shoulder is a common examination to assess for rotator cuff tears or impingement. Supraspinatus is the most common muscle involved in these pathologies and this MRI nicely demonstrates the relatively narrow subacromial space. Impingement occurs if:

- the subacromial space becomes further narrowed
- there is enlargement of the supraspinatus muscle.

The clavicle may be used as a horizontal margin to differentiate between the trapezius and deltoid muscles on shoulder MRI:

- trapezius lies superior to the clavicle
- deltoid is inferior to the clavicle.

Case 8.8

A Bladder

B Peripheral zone of prostate

C Right levator ani muscle

D Central zone of prostate

E Left obturator internus muscle

The zonal anatomy of the prostate is well demonstrated in the coronal plane. In addition, the verumontanum is seen centrally as an area of low signal with a midline high signal vertical line. It signifies the opening of the ejaculatory ducts in the prostatic urethra and is Latin for 'mountain ridge'.

The anatomy of the levator ani muscles can be appreciated as they insert into the perineal body, a fibrous node posterior to the male urethra or the urethra and vagina in females.

The obturator internus fibres are located lateral to the levator ani group. The muscle originates from the anterolateral walls of the pelvis and covers the obturator foramen. It travels inferiorly, through the lesser sciatic foramen, to insert into the greater trochanter of the femur.

Case 8.9

A Right vertebral artery

B Right posterior inferior cerebellar artery

C Right superior cerebellar artery

D Interpeduncular segment of the left posterior cerebral artery (PCA)

E Ambient segment of the right PCA

The first step in approaching a DSA angiogram is recognising a main vessel and then determining its branches. The vertebrobasilar circulation resembles a 'tree' on DSA angiography.

On the frontal projection, it looks like a 'tree on a windless day' (**Figure 8.1**), whereas on the lateral projection, it is shaped like a 'tree on a windy day' (see Figure 5.1, p. 242).

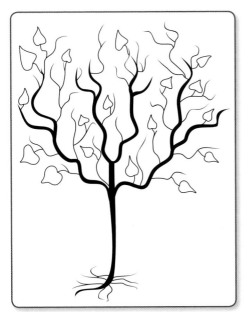

Figure 8.1 'Tree on a windless day', resembling the vertebrobasilar circulation on frontal DSA angiography.

The posterior cerebral arteries (PCA) are the terminal branches of the basilar artery. Each PCA has three segments:

- **P1** – interpeduncular (pre-communicating) segment between basilar bifurcation and the origin of the posterior communicating artery
- **P2** – ambient segment, which runs around the brainstem in the ambient cistern
- **P3** – quadrigeminal segment, which extends from the quadrigeminal plate to the calcarine fissure.

Case 8.10

A Cricoid cartilage of larynx

B Right lobe of thyroid gland

C Right common carotid artery

D Left internal jugular vein

E Left vertebral artery

The thyroid and cricoid cartilages are parts of the larynx. The thyroid gland is high attenuation on CT due to its high iodine content. The vertebral arteries can be identified by their paired prevertebral locations. The common carotid arteries usually bifurcate at the upper end of the thyroid cartilage (C4 level) into internal and external carotid arteries.

Case 8.11

A Right serratus anterior muscle

B Left hepatic vein

C Distal oesophagus

D Aorta

E Body of T10

The relationship of the aorta posterior to the oesophagus is well seen. Just lateral to this, the azygos and hemiazygos venous systems are visible. It is important to be able to recognise the anatomical levels of significant structures such as the gastro-oesophageal junction. Questions may ask you to identify the axial level for each image.

Further important levels include: entry of aorta, IVC and oesophagus through the diaphragm. An aide-mémoire to help memorise these levels is listed below:

Aortic hiatus = 12 letters = T12

Oesophagus = 10 letters = T10

Vena cava = 8 letters = T8

Case 8.12

  A Transverse colon

  B Sigmoid colon

  C Right ischial spine

  D Right anterior inferior iliac spine

  E Piriformis

The sacrospinous ligament is attached laterally to the ischial spine and medially to the lateral aspects of the sacrum and coccyx, lying anterior to (and merging with) the sacrotuberous ligament. These two ligaments help form the boundaries of the greater and lesser sciatic foramina. The ischial spine also has muscular attachments (for coccygeus, levator ani and gemellus superior). It forms an important landmark for pudendal nerve blocks in obstetric anaesthesia.

Rectus femoris is attached to the anterior inferior iliac spine, whereas sartorius is attached to the anterior superior iliac spine – knowledge of these attachments is important in both examinations and in real life scenarios since avulsion injuries are not infrequent. Remember – SartoriuS – aSiS; rectus FEmoris – anterior inFErior iliac spine.

Case 8.13

  A Left ventricle

  B Papillary muscle

  C Left atrium

  D Spinal cord (thoracic)

  E Anterior leaflet of mitral valve

This is an oblique coronal view of the left ventricle in which the mitral valve, left atrium and ventricle are seen in profile. The thoracic spinal cord is seen, surrounded by CSF.

Orientation on an oblique view can be difficult and in this image, it is worth appreciating that the left atrium is the most posterior chamber, adjacent to the spine. This helps identify the left ventricle and the mitral valve. It is also worth noting that the blood returns high signal (bright blood sequence) unlike standard sequences in which a flow void is noted.

Case 8.14

  A Right mastoid air cells

  B Foramen magnum

  C Left zygomatic arch

  D Left mandibular ramus

  E Right mandibular body

The mandible is the strongest of all the facial bones. It consists of two hemimandibles which are fused anteriorly in the midline at the mental symphysis. Each hemimandible contains the following portions:

- The horizontally curved body
- The vertically orientated ramus, which unites with the ipsilateral body to form a right angle (*angle of mandible*)
- Three processes:
  - **Condylar process** – superoposterior projection of the ramus, part of the temporomandibular joint
  - **Coronoid process** – superoanterior projection of the ramus, insertion of the temporalis muscle
  - **Alveolar process** – tooth-bearing area of the mandible.

Case 8.15

A Right rectus abdominis muscle

B Left external oblique muscle

C Left internal oblique muscle

D Left transversus abdominis muscle

E Left erector spinae muscles

The abdominal wall can be divided into three parts – anterior, lateral and posterior. Each part of the abdominal wall comprises the following layers (from deep to superficial):

- the extraperitoneal fat
- the parietal peritoneum
- the fascial layer – the name of which is derived from the structures it covers. In the anterior abdominal wall it is called the fascia transversalis.
- the muscular layer – which is not present in the posterior abdominal wall
- the subcutaneous fat layer
- the superficial fascia
- the skin.

The muscular layer of the anterior and lateral abdominal wall consists of four muscles, which lead into the fibrous linea alba in the midline:

- paired paramedian rectus abdominis muscles, forming the most anterior wall
- three muscles forming each of the anterolateral walls, from superficial to deep:
  - external oblique muscle
  - internal oblique muscle
  - transversus abdominis muscle

Each of these muscles can be separately identified on abdominal CT or MRI due to the presence of intermuscular fat and connective tissue. They originate from the lower lateral ribs and their aponeuroses terminate in the inguinal regions, where they form the inguinal ligaments.

Case 8.16

A Right distal fibula

B Right talus

C Right navicular

D Right cuboid

E Base of the fifth right metatarsal

The calcaneum, talus and cuboid begin to ossify in utero. The cuneiform ossification centres develop at one to three years of age (progressing in the order lateral, intermediate and finally medial cuneiform). Ossification of the navicular commences in the third year of life, sometimes with several ossification centres apparent. Accordingly, of all the ossification centres visible on this radiograph of a 3-year-old child, the navicular ossification centre is the least well developed. Metatarsal and phalangeal shaft ossification centres also start to develop in utero, although ossification centres of the phalangeal epiphyses are usually not seen until after the age of 2, and the ossification centres of the metatarsal bases are typically evident after the age of 3 years.

Case 8.17

A Right gluteus maximus

B Left rectus abdominis

C Greater trochanter of the left femur

D Right iliacus

E Left sacroiliac joint

Three gluteal muscles make up the buttocks and comprise (from deep to superficial):

1. gluteus minimus

2. gluteus medius

3. gluteus maximus

Gluteus medius and minimus insert into the ipsilateral greater trochanter of the femur. Gluteus maximus has a combined insertion into the iliotibial band/tract and the gluteal tuberosity of the femur.

Case 8.18

A Pinna of the right ear

B Epitympanum

C Scutum

D Manubrium of the malleus

E Tympanic membrane

The middle ear (tympanic) cavity is divided into three compartments (epitympanum, mesotympanum and hypotympanum) by lines drawn along the superior and inferior margins of the external auditory meatus.

The roof (tegmen tympani) separates the tympanic cavity and the middle cranial fossa. The scutum is a prominence at the lateral wall of the epitympanum to which the tympanic membrane attaches.

The auditory ossicles: malleus, incus and stapes articulate with each other in that order (from lateral to medial).

Case 8.19

A Left lamina of the thyroid cartilage

B Anterior tubercle of C5

C Right vertebral artery

D Right lamina of C5

E Bilateral double foramina transversaria

The foramen transversarium is present on each side in each of the upper six cervical vertebrae (not C7), with the vertebral artery passing through it as it courses superiorly to form the basilar artery with its contralateral counterpart. Double foramina transversaria are a recognised anatomical variant and may be present unilaterally or bilaterally, as in this case.

Case 8.20

A Right lobe of liver

B Portal vein

C Hepatic artery

D Common bile duct

E Hepatopetal (towards the liver)

This is the classic view used to visualise structures at porta hepatis. The round hepatic artery (visualised in transverse section) is seen to be sandwiched between the portal vein and common bile duct (visualised in longitudinal section).

Chapter 9

Mock paper 9

20 cases to be answered in 75 minutes

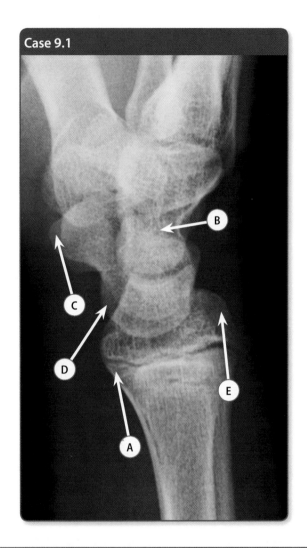

Case 9.1

QUESTION		WRITE YOUR ANSWER HERE
A	Name the structure labelled A.	
B	Name the structure labelled B.	
C	Name the structure labelled C.	
D	Name the structure labelled D.	
E	Name the structure labelled E.	

Case 9.2

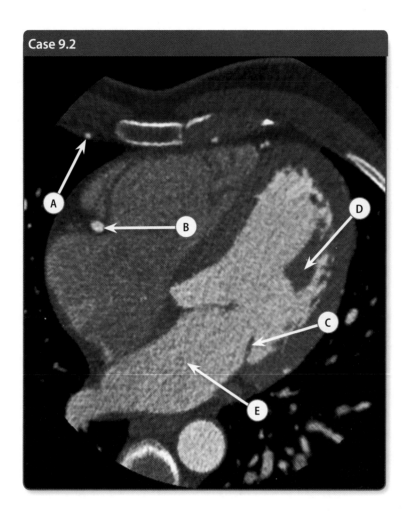

Case 9.2

QUESTION		WRITE YOUR ANSWER HERE
A	Name the structure labelled A.	
B	Name the structure labelled B.	
C	Name the structure labelled C.	
D	Name the structure labelled D.	
E	Name the chamber labelled E.	

Case 9.3

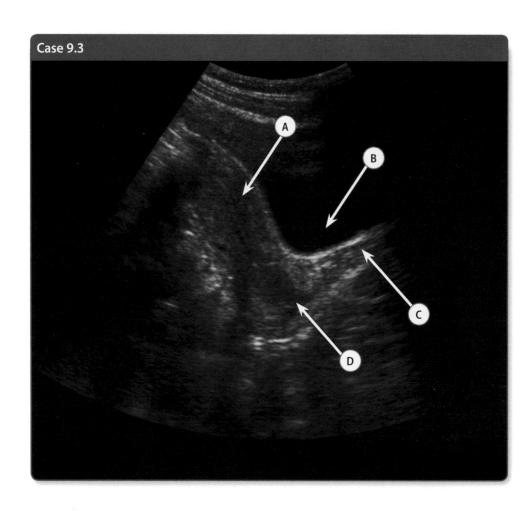

Case 9.3

	QUESTION	WRITE YOUR ANSWER HERE
A	Name the structure labelled A.	
B	Name the structure labelled B.	
C	Name the structure labelled C.	
D	Name the structure labelled D.	
E	During which phase of the menstrual cycle will the endometrium be thickest?	

Case 9.4

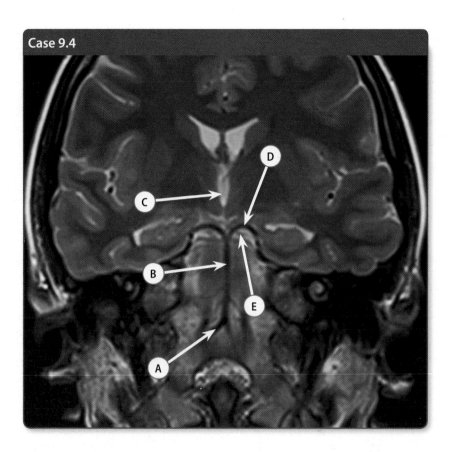

Case 9.4

QUESTION		WRITE YOUR ANSWER HERE
A	Name the structure labelled A.	
B	Name the structure labelled B.	
C	Name the structure labelled C	
D	Name the structure labelled D.	
E	Name the neural structure labelled E.	

Case 9.5

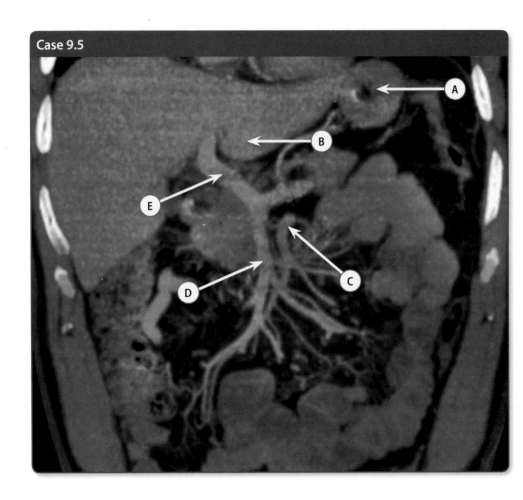

Case 9.5

QUESTION		WRITE YOUR ANSWER HERE
A	Name the structure labelled A.	
B	Name the structure labelled B.	
C	Name the structure labelled C.	
D	Name the structure labelled D.	
E	Name the structure labelled E.	

Case 9.6

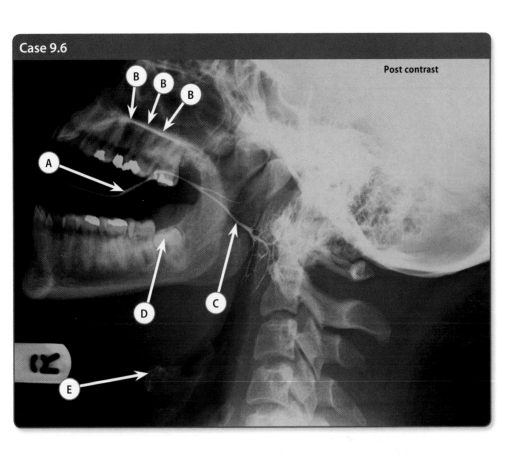

Post contrast

Case 9.6

QUESTION		WRITE YOUR ANSWER HERE
A	Name the non-anatomical structure labelled A.	
B	Name the structure labelled B.	
C	Where does the structure labelled C drain into?	
D	Name the structure labelled D.	
E	Name the structure labelled E.	

Case 9.7

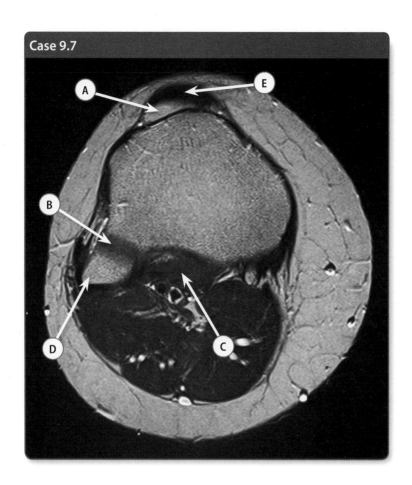

Case 9.7

	QUESTION	WRITE YOUR ANSWER HERE
A	Name the structure labelled A.	
B	Name the structure labelled B.	
C	Name the structure labelled C.	
D	Name the structure labelled D.	
E	Name the distal insertion site for the structure labelled E.	

Case 9.8

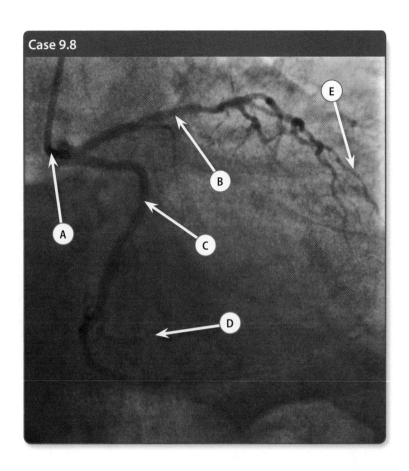

Case 9.8

QUESTION		WRITE YOUR ANSWER HERE
A	Name the structure labelled A.	
B	Name the structure labelled B.	
C	Name the structure labelled C.	
D	Name the structure labelled D.	
E	Name the structure labelled E.	

Case 9.9

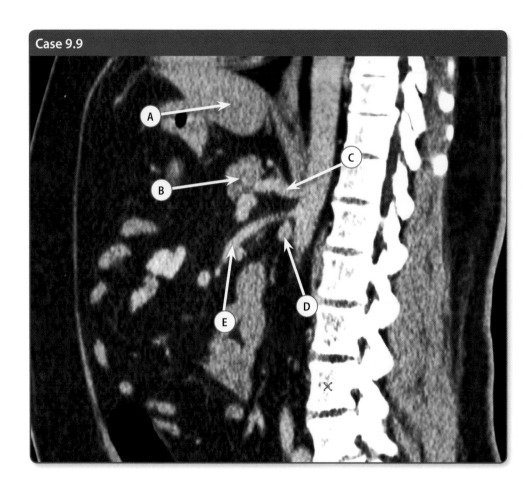

Case 9.9

QUESTION		WRITE YOUR ANSWER HERE
A	Name the structure labelled A.	
B	Name the structure labelled B.	
C	Name the structure labelled C.	
D	Name the structure labelled D.	
E	Name the structure labelled E.	

Case 9.10

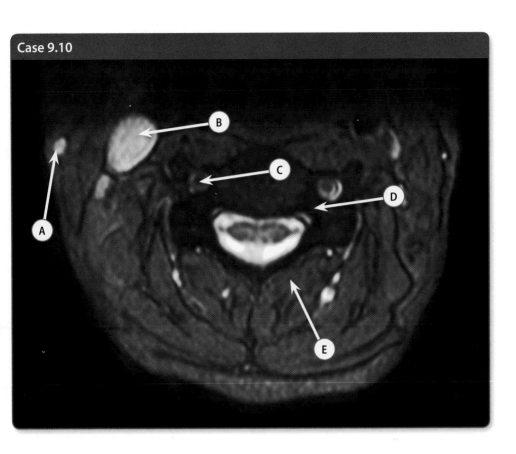

Case 9.10 Axial MRI at the level of C5

QUESTION		WRITE YOUR ANSWER HERE
A	Name the structure labelled A.	
B	Name the structure labelled B.	
C	Name the structure labelled C.	
D	Name the structure labelled D.	
E	Name the structure labelled E.	

Case 9.11

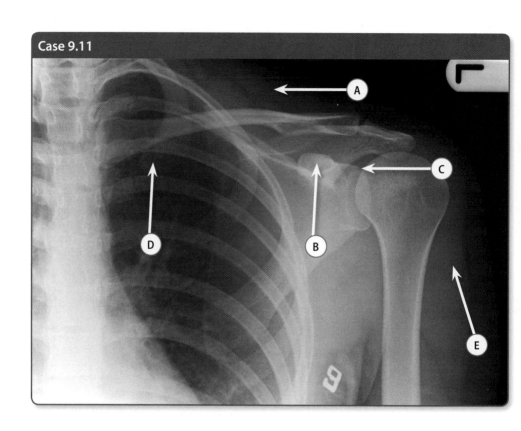

Case 9.11

QUESTION		WRITE YOUR ANSWER HERE
A	Name the structure labelled A.	
B	Name the muscle that inserts into the structure labelled B.	
C	Name the muscle that originates from the structure labelled C.	
D	Name the structure labelled D.	
E	Name the structure labelled E.	

Case 9.12

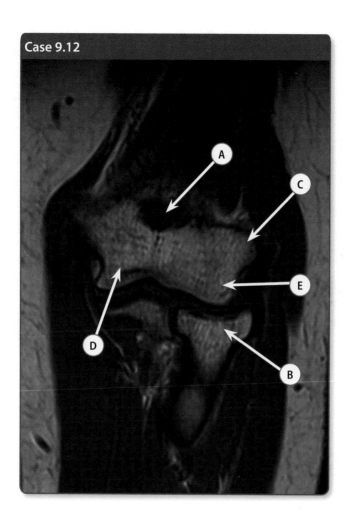

Case 9.12

QUESTION		WRITE YOUR ANSWER HERE
A	Name the structure labelled A.	
B	Name the structure labelled B.	
C	Name the structure that originates from C.	
D	Name the structure labelled D.	
E	Name the structure labelled E.	

Case 9.13

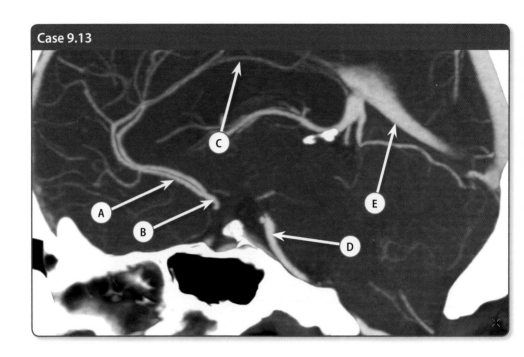

Case 9.13

QUESTION		WRITE YOUR ANSWER HERE
A	Name the structure labelled A.	
B	Name the structure labelled B.	
C	Name the structure labelled C.	
D	Name the structure labelled D.	
E	Name the structure labelled E.	

Case 9.14

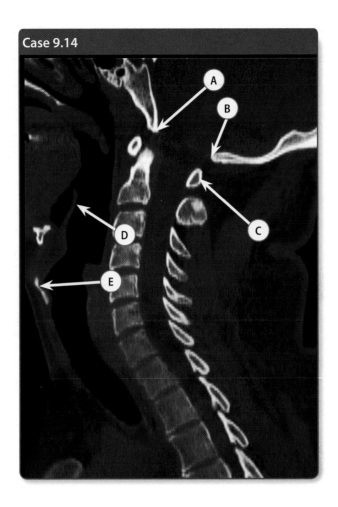

Case 9.14

QUESTION		WRITE YOUR ANSWER HERE
A	Name the structure labelled A.	
B	Name the structure labelled B.	
C	Name the structure labelled C.	
D	Name the structure labelled D.	
E	Name the structure labelled E.	

Case 9.15

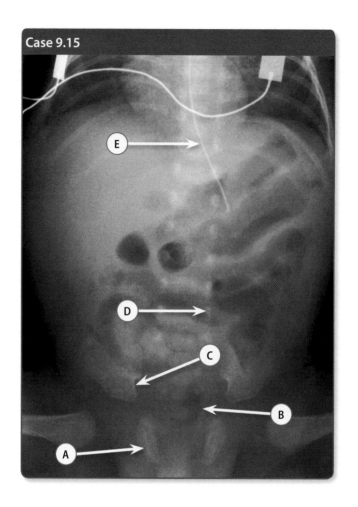

Case 9.15

QUESTION		WRITE YOUR ANSWER HERE
A	Name the structure labelled A.	
B	In which structure does gas labelled B lie?	
C	Name the line labelled C.	
D	Name the structure labelled D.	
E	Name the tube labelled E.	

Case 9.16

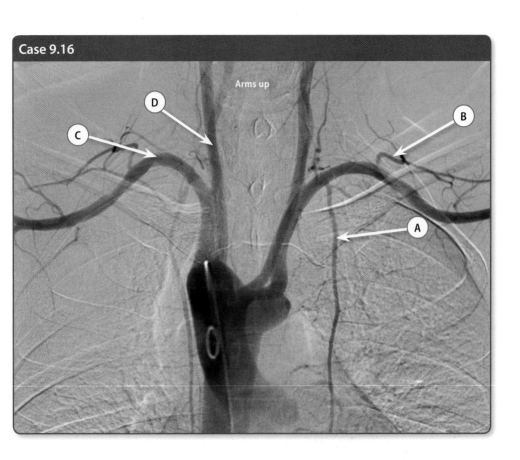

Case 9.16

QUESTION		WRITE YOUR ANSWER HERE
A	Name the structure labelled A.	
B	Name the structure labelled B.	
C	Name the structure labelled C.	
D	Name the structure labelled D.	
E	Which anatomical variant is present on this image?	

Case 9.17

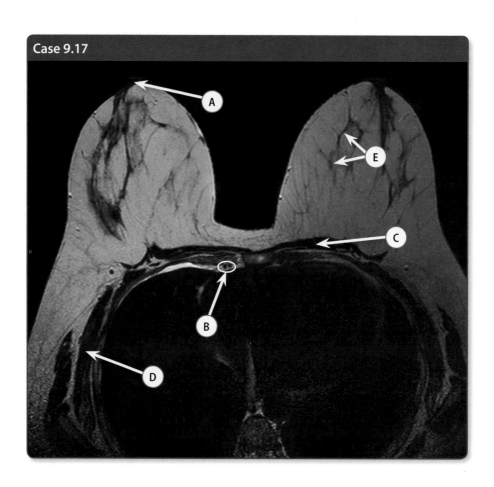

Case 9.17

QUESTION		WRITE YOUR ANSWER HERE
A	Name the structure labelled A.	
B	Name the structure labelled B.	
C	Name the structure labelled C.	
D	Name the structure labelled D.	
E	Name the structure labelled E.	

Case 9.18

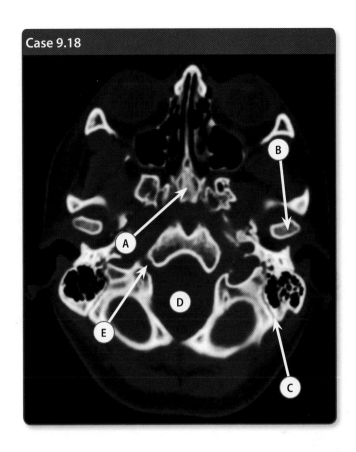

Case 9.18

QUESTION	WRITE YOUR ANSWER HERE
A Name the structure labelled A.	
B Name the structure labelled B.	
C Name the structure labelled C.	
D Name the structure labelled D.	
E Which cranial nerve exits the cranial cavity via the foramen labelled E?	

Case 9.19

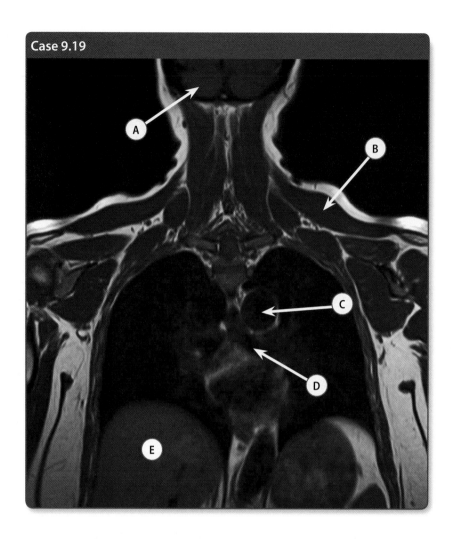

Case 9.19

QUESTION		WRITE YOUR ANSWER HERE
A	Name the structure labelled A.	
B	Name the structure labelled B.	
C	Name the structure labelled C.	
D	Name the structure labelled D.	
E	Name the structure labelled E.	

Case 9.20

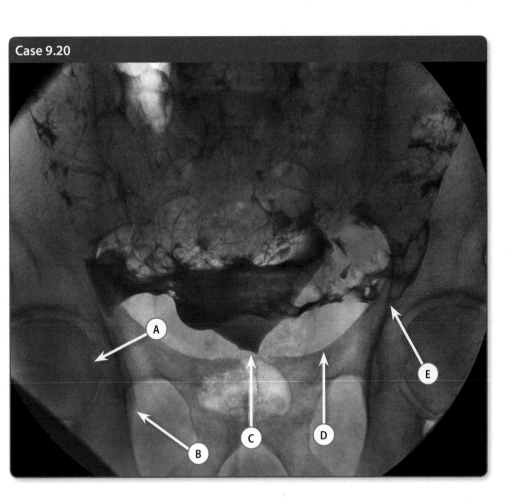

Case 9.20

QUESTION		WRITE YOUR ANSWER HERE
A	Name the structure labelled A.	
B	Name the structure labelled B.	
C	Name the structure that is causing the impression labelled C.	
D	Name the osseous line labelled D.	
E	Which artery courses within this peritoneal reflection?	

Answers

Case 9.1

A Anterior corner of the distal metaphysis of the radius

B Capitate

C Distal pole of the scaphoid

D Lunate

E Epiphysis of distal radius

An important feature to appreciate on the lateral radiograph of the wrist is the contiguity of the distal radius, lunate, capitate and third metacarpal, which should lie in a straight line.

If the lunate is disrupted from the line, the diagnosis of a lunate dislocation should be made.

If the radiolunate line is preserved but the line no longer passes through the capitate, a perilunate dislocation is likely.

Case 9.2

A Right internal mammary/internal thoracic artery

B Right coronary artery

C Posterior leaflet of the mitral valve

D Papillary muscle

E Left atrium

High resolution cardiac CT scans nicely depict the coronary anatomy. In addition, anatomy of the cardiac valves, chambers and other intrinsic cardiac structures are visible.

The internal mammary arteries are important, particularly the left, if an internal mammary bypass is being considered.

On the current image, the mitral valve – the only bicuspid valve – is evident. The aortic, pulmonary and tricuspid valves all have three cusps.

Case 9.3

A Fundus of the uterus

B Urinary bladder

C Vagina

D Uterine cervix

E Secretory phase

Endometrial thickness varies with the menopausal state of the patient and, if pre-menopausal, with the stage of the menstrual cycle. The endometrium is evident as an echogenic stripe on longitudinal ultrasonography, surrounded by hypoechoic myometrium. The vagina is a posterior relation of the bladder and can also be seen as an echogenic stripe which lies at an angle to the body of the uterus.

Case 9.4

A Right vertebral artery

B Basilar artery

C Third ventricle

D Left posterior cerebral artery

E Left oculomotor nerve

This is a standard view for the visualisation of the cisternal portion of the oculomotor nerve. The characteristic shape of the vascular structures resembles a 'man in glasses', as depicted in **Figure 9.1**, with oculomotor nerves being eyes, posterior cerebral arteries and superior cerebellar arteries forming glasses, basilar artery as body, anterior inferior cerebellar arteries as hands and vertebral arteries as legs of the man.

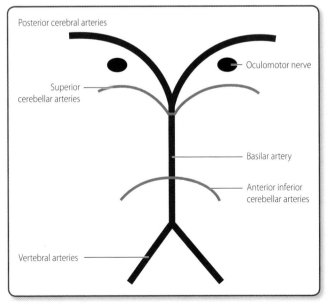

Figure 9.1 'Man in glasses' schematic illustration of the characteristic shape of posterior circulation vessels and their relation to the oculomotor nerve.

Case 9.5

A Stomach

B Left lobe of liver

C Superior mesenteric artery

D Superior mesenteric vein

E Portal vein

The portal vein is formed by the confluence of the superior mesenteric vein and the splenic vein. The superior mesenteric vein lies to the right of the superior mesenteric artery and posterior to the pancreas. Note that there is a small amount of gas in the stomach and scattered throughout the large bowel, whereas the small bowel (shown on the left side of the abdomen), contains no gas. These are normal appearances.

Case 9.6

A Catheter with contrast

B Palatine process of maxilla

C Oral vestibule opposite to the second upper molar tooth

D Crown of unerupted right inferior third molar tooth (right lower eighth tooth)

E Body of the hyoid bone

There are three paired major salivary glands: parotid, submandibular and sublingual. Of these, the parotid and submandibular are investigated most frequently by sialography. **Table 9.1** will help to distinguish between them.

Be aware that the arrow may point not only at anatomical structures, but also at various devices visible on the radiograph, such as the catheter used to cannulate the parotid duct and contrast injection in this case.

Table 9.1 Characteristic features of main salivary glands

	Parotid gland	Submandibular gland
Location	Superficial and posterior to the ramus of the mandible	Lies inferior to the mandible, between the body of the mandible and hyoid bone
Main duct	Duct of Stensen: emerges from the gland anteriorly	Duct of Wharton: emerges from the gland superoanteriorly
Drainage	Papilla in the oral vestibule opposite to the second upper molar tooth	Papilla on the floor of the buccal cavity

Case 9.7

  A Hoffa's (infrapatellar) fat pad

  B Proximal tibiofibular joint

  C Popliteus muscle

  D Head of fibula

  E Tibial tuberosity

This question has been purposefully constructed to aid in actual examination technique.

1. Identify the anatomical region of the image – the proximal tibiofibular joint is visualised, thus allowing you to be confident that you are below the level of the patella, enabling you to answer B/D.

2. E – the structure returns low signal suggestive of tendinous origin. From point 1, you know that the image is below the patella – this should make you think of the patellar tendon which attaches to the tibial tuberosity.

3. A – this structure demonstrates isointense signal relative to fatty marrow and the subcutaneous fat. It is bounded by the tibial cortex posteriorly and the patellar tendon anteriorly. Remember, the image is below the level of the patella, hence you should think of Hoffa's fat pad.

4. C – the popliteus muscle originates from the lateral femoral condyle and inserts into the posteromedial tibia, thus crossing the midline of the joint anterior to the posterior tibial vessels.

Case 9.8

  A Left mainstem coronary artery

  B Left anterior descending branch

  C Left circumflex artery

  D Obtuse marginal branch

  E Diagonal branch

The left main coronary artery arises from the left coronary sinus and gives rise to the left anterior descending artery and the left circumflex coronary artery. In up to 15 % of cases, a third branch arises at the bifurcation: the intermediate artery.

Case 9.9

  A Left lobe of the liver

  B Body of pancreas

  C Coeliac axis/trunk

D Left renal vein

E Superior mesenteric artery

Three unpaired branches of the abdominal aorta arise from the anterior wall of the aorta between the L1 and L3 vertebral levels:

- the coeliac axis/trunk at the superior margin of L1 vertebra level
- the superior mesenteric artery (SMA) at the level of the mid-body of L1 vertebrae
- the inferior mesenteric artery (IMA) at L3 level.

It is important to note the relationship between two of these three major abdominal arterial vessels and adjacent viscera, which is clearly demonstrated on this sagittal midline view. The coeliac axis lies posterosuperior to the body of pancreas and the SMA runs anterior to the left renal vein. Inferior to the SMA trunk lies the third part of the duodenum, which can be compressed between the SMA and the vertebral column in very thin individuals or after rapid weight loss in a condition known as a nutcracker syndrome.

Case 9.10

A Right external jugular vein

B Right internal jugular vein

C Right vertebral artery

D Left pedicle of C5

E Left erector spinae muscle

This is an axial STIR (short tau inversion recovery) MRI at the level of C5. STIR MRI sequences have a dual role to play in imaging of the spine, by improving detection of both vertebral metastatic disease and intramedullary disease of the spinal cord. As seen in this image, there is good anatomical detail of the spinal cord, with clear differentiation between grey matter (central) and white matter (peripheral). Blood vessels are also clearly demonstrated.

Case 9.11

A Left trapezius muscle

B Left pectoralis minor muscle

C Left long head of biceps brachii muscle

D Left anterior first rib

E Left deltoid muscle

It is important to differentiate the origin and insertion of muscles, which is key to answering (B) and (C) correctly.

The coracoid process serves as the:

- origin of coracobrachialis and short head of biceps brachii
- insertion for pectoralis minor

The origin of the long head of biceps brachii muscle is the supraglenoid tubercle. Insertion is into the ipsilateral radial tuberosity.

Although plain radiographs are not a conventional means of examining musculature, this example demonstrates the trapezius and deltoid muscles nicely outlined by less dense fat.

Case 9.12

A Coronoid fossa of the humerus

B Head of radius

C Common extensor tendon

D Trochlea of the humerus

E Capitulum of the humerus

Key osseous anatomy of the distal humerus includes:

1. capitulum – articulates with the head of radius
2. trochlea – lies within the trochlear notch of the proximal ulna
3. medial epicondyle – origin of common flexor tendon
4. lateral epicondyle – origin of common extensor tendon.

Case 9.13

A A2 (post-communicating) segment of the anterior cerebral artery (ACA)

B A1 (pre-communicating) segment of the ACA

C Pericallosal artery

D Basilar artery

E Straight venous sinus

The ACA is a terminal branch of the internal carotid artery and is divided into three segments:

A1 – pre-communicating (horizontal) segment which gives off the anterior communicating artery (A-com)

A2 – post-communicating segment which extends from A-com to the bifurcation and divides into the callosomarginal and pericallosal arteries

A3 – pericallosal artery – terminal branch of ACA which extends posteriorly in the pericallosal sulcus

A4 – callosomarginal artery – present in only 60% of cases running anteriorly from the bifurcation.

Case 9.14

A Basion

B Opisthion

C Posterior arch of C1 vertebra

D Epiglottis

E Thyroid cartilage

Foramen magnum is an opening in the occipital bone and the largest aperture of the skull base. Its lateral borders are formed by the occipital condyles, which form part of the craniocervical junction. Anteriorly, it is bounded by the basilar part of the occipital bone, the middle and most inferiorly projected point of which is called the basion. Posteriorly, it is bounded by the squama occipitalis, the midpoint of which is called the opisthion. The basion and opisthion are used as cephalometric and anatomical landmarks.

Case 9.15

A Right ischium

B Rectum

C Right iliopectineal line

D Left pedicle of L4

E Nasogastric tube

Anatomical detail on abdominal radiographs in neonatal and paediatric patients is often limited in comparison with adult patients. Accordingly, questions relating to this area are more likely to focus on osseous anatomy, or on lines and tubes that may be present on the radiograph. A nasogastric tube is shown here, but umbilical arterial and venous catheters (UAC and UVC) also typically feature on neonatal radiographs. These can be differentiated as follows: the UAC takes a characteristic inferior dip in the pelvis as it enters the iliac arteries, whereas the UVC travels in a cephalad direction throughout.

Case 9.16

A Left internal mammary artery

B Left costocervical trunk

C Right subclavian artery

D Right common carotid artery

E Double aortic arch (DAA)

A DAA is the most frequent form of vascular ring. DAA may surround the trachea and oesophagus and hence may cause compression of these structures. If the compression is severe, symptoms such as dyspnoea, recurrent pneumonia, stridor, dysphagia, and feeding difficulties may be observed at birth. However, when compression is minimal, DAA can remain undiagnosed until adulthood.

Embryologically, the ventral and dorsal aortas are connected by aortic arches which persist or involute to give rise to the normal aortic arch, its branches and minor arteries of the head. The right fourth aortic arch normally involutes at about 36–38 days and the left fourth aortic arch persists to give rise to the normal left aortic arch. The persistence of both the right and left fourth aortic arches leads to a double aortic arch.

Incidence of congenital heart disease in patients with DAA has been reported to be as high as 20%, the most common being the tetralogy of Fallot and transposition of great vessels.

Case 9.17

A Right nipple

B Right internal mammary/internal thoracic vessels

C Left pectoralis major muscle

D Right serratus anterior muscle

E Suspensory ligaments

MRI of the breast shows anatomical structures such as blood vessels, lymph nodes, suspensory ligaments and underlying muscular structures with great detail. Be sure to take this into consideration as a question such as this one will also likely yield questions not related to breast anatomy.

The proportion of breast tissue can vary widely and usually decreases with age, a concept known as age-related involutional change.

Case 9.18

A Vomer

B Left mandibular condyle

C Left occipitomastoid suture

D Medulla oblongata

E Left hypoglossal nerve (CN XII)

The occipital bone contains two important foramina – foramen magnum and the hypoglossal canal.

Foramen magnum is the largest opening of the skull base, connecting the posterior fossa and the spinal canal.

 The contents of foramen magnum include the following:

- Medulla oblongata
- Vertebral artery and vein
- Spinal accessory nerve (CN XI)

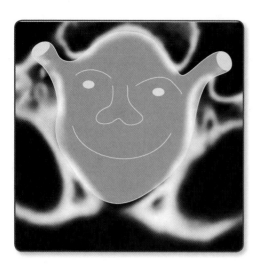

Figure 9.2 Schematic illustration of the relationship between foramen magnum and the hypoglossal canal resembling the head of Shrek.

The hypoglossal canal transmits the hypoglossal nerve, which innervates the extrinsic muscles of the tongue. On the axial CT images, the hypoglossal canals are evident adjacent to the anterolateral borders of foramen magnum and posterior to the clivus. Together with foramen magnum, they resemble the head of Shrek (the famous computer-animated character), as depicted in **Figure 9.2**.

Case 9.19

A Right cerebellar hemisphere

B Left trapezius muscle

C Arch of the aorta

D Left main bronchus

E Right lobe of liver

The trapezius is a large fan-shaped muscle. Its superior fibres arise from: the external occipital protuberance; the superior nuchal line of the occipital bone; and ligamentum nuchae. From these origins they pass inferolaterally to insert into the posterior border of the lateral third of the clavicle.

The middle fibres of the trapezius arise from the spinous process of the C7 and the spinous processes of the upper three thoracic vertebrae. They insert into the medial margin of the acromion.

The inferior fibres arise from the spinous processes of the remaining thoracic vertebrae (T4–T12) and pass superolaterally, converging near the scapula to insert into a tubercle at the apex of the spine of the scapula.

In addition to the anatomical structures of the chest, the brain stem and upper abdominal organs are visible and should routinely be scrutinised for the presence of incidental pathology.

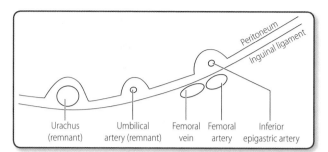

Figure 9.3 Peritoneal reflections at the level of the umbilical ligament.

Peritoneum
Inguinal ligament

| Urachus (remnant) | Umbilical artery (remnant) | Femoral vein | Femoral artery | Inferior epigastric artery |

Case 9.20

A Fovea of the right femoral head

B Right ischial spine

C Median umbilical fold

D Left iliopectineal line

E Left inferior epigastric artery

This is an example of a herniogram, with contrast injected into the peritoneal cavity. The outlines of the peritoneal reflections in the anterior pelvis are illustrated in **Figure 9.3**. Inguinal herniae medial to the epigastric artery are of the direct type and laterally-sited herniae are of the indirect type. **Figure 9.3** shows the peritoneal reflections at the level of the umbilical ligament. The lateral umbilical fold is formed by the inferior epigastric artery, which is closely related to the deep inguinal ring and its contents.

Chapter 10

Mock paper 10

20 cases to be answered in 75 minutes

Case 10.1

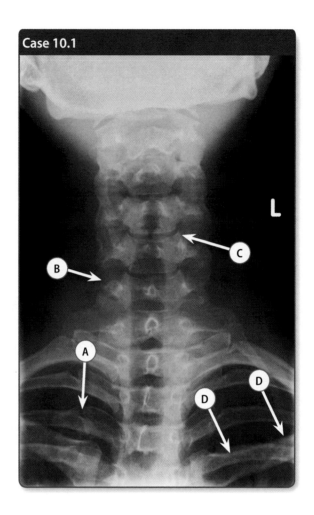

Case 10.1

QUESTION		WRITE YOUR ANSWER HERE
A	Name the joint labelled A.	
B	Name the structure labelled B.	
C	Name the structure labelled C.	
D	Name the structure labelled D.	
E	Which anatomical variant is present on this image?	

Case 10.2

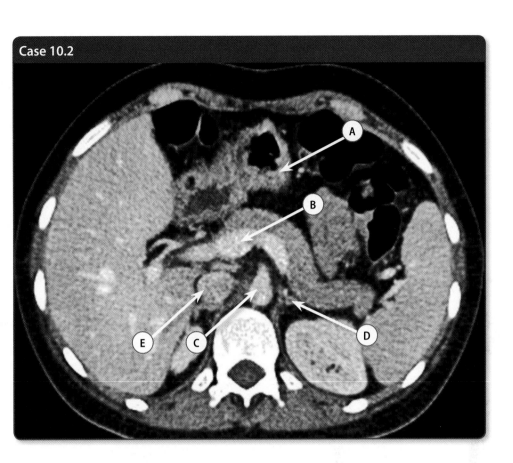

Case 10.2

QUESTION		WRITE YOUR ANSWER HERE
A	Name the structure labelled A.	
B	Name the structure labelled B.	
C	Name the structure labelled C.	
D	Name the structure labelled D.	
E	Name the structure labelled E.	

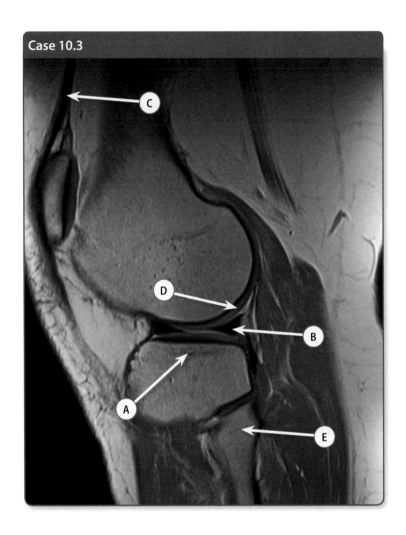

Case 10.3

Case 10.3	
QUESTION	**WRITE YOUR ANSWER HERE**
A Name the structure labelled A.	
B Name the structure labelled B.	
C Name the structure labelled C.	
D Name the structure labelled D.	
E Name the structure labelled E.	

Case 10.4

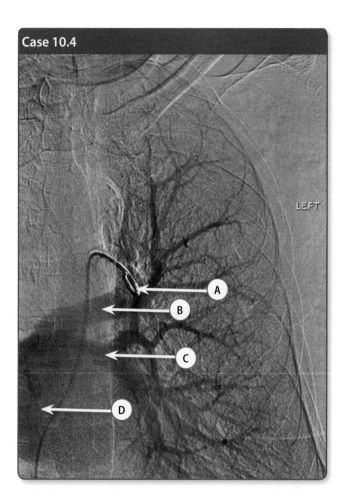

Case 10.4		
QUESTION		**WRITE YOUR ANSWER HERE**
A	Where is the catheter tip located at position A?	
B	Name the structure labelled B.	
C	Name the structure labelled C.	
D	Name the structure labelled D.	
E	How many pulmonary veins are normally present?	

Case 10.5

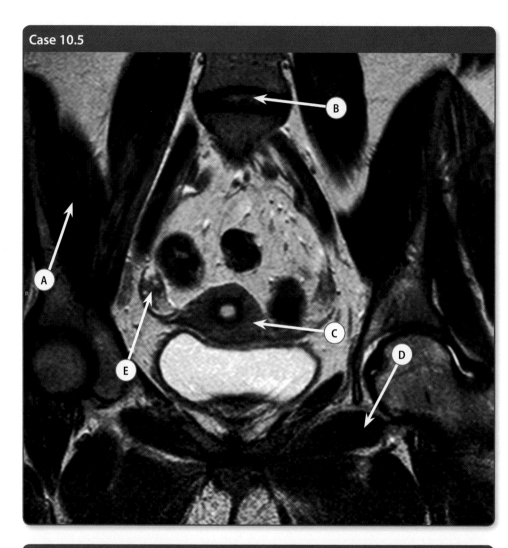

Case 10.5

QUESTION		WRITE YOUR ANSWER HERE
A	Name the structure labelled A.	
B	Name the structure labelled B.	
C	Name the structure labelled C.	
D	Name the structure labelled D.	
E	Name the structure labelled E.	

Case 10.6

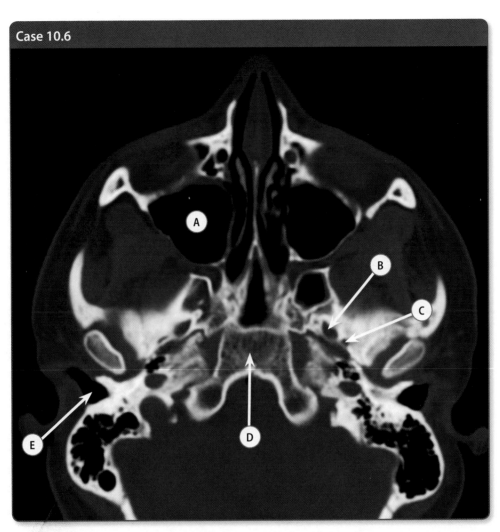

Case 10.6

QUESTION		WRITE YOUR ANSWER HERE
A	Name the structure labelled A.	
B	Which cranial nerve exits the cranium via the foramen labelled B?	
C	Name the structure labelled C.	
D	Name the structure labelled D.	
E	Name the structure labelled E.	

Case 10.7

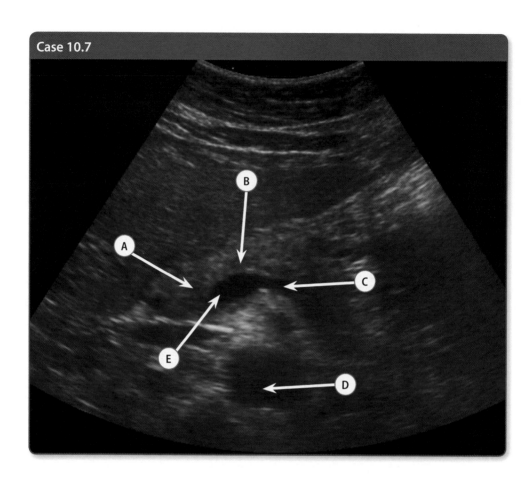

Case 10.7

QUESTION		WRITE YOUR ANSWER HERE
A	Name the structure labelled A.	
B	Name the structure labelled B.	
C	Name the structure labelled C.	
D	Name the structure labelled D.	
E	Name the structure labelled E.	

Case 10.8

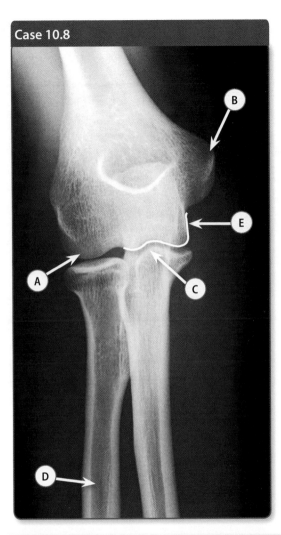

Case 10.8

QUESTION		WRITE YOUR ANSWER HERE
A	Name the structure labelled A.	
B	What originates from the structure labelled B.	
C	Name the structure labelled C.	
D	Name the structure labelled D.	
E	Name the structure that is outlined and labelled E.	

Case 10.9

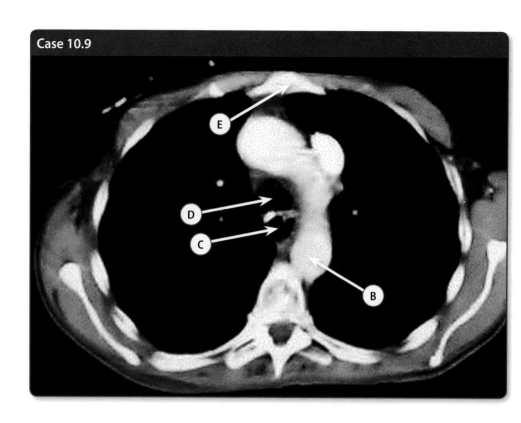

Case 10.9

QUESTION		WRITE YOUR ANSWER HERE
A	Which anatomical variant is present on this image?	
B	Name the structure labelled B.	
C	Name the structure labelled C.	
D	Name the structure labelled D.	
E	Name the structure labelled E.	

Case 10.10

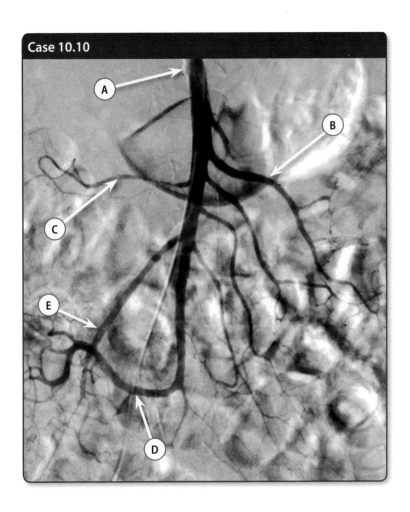

Case 10.10

QUESTION		WRITE YOUR ANSWER HERE
A	Name the structure labelled A.	
B	Name the structure labelled B.	
C	Name the structure labelled C.	
D	Name the structure labelled D.	
E	Name the structure labelled E.	

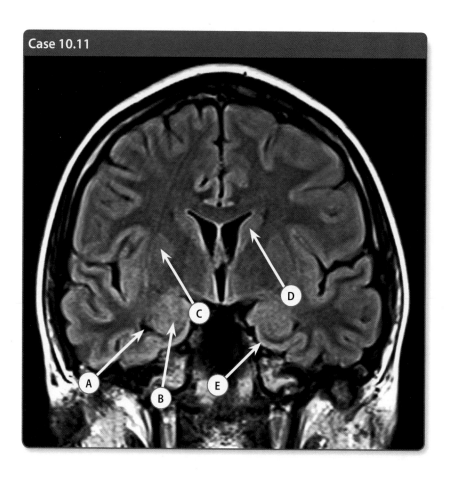

Case 10.11

Case 10.11

QUESTION		WRITE YOUR ANSWER HERE
A	Name the structure labelled A.	
B	Name the structure labelled B.	
C	Name the structure labelled C.	
D	Name the structure labelled D.	
E	Name the gyrus labelled E.	

Case 10.12

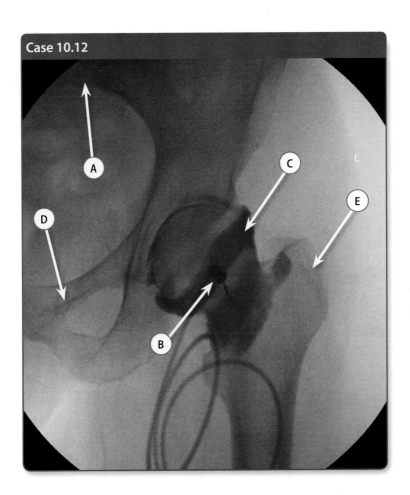

Case 10.12

QUESTION		WRITE YOUR ANSWER HERE
A	Name the structure labelled A.	
B	What is the radio-opaque non-anatomical structure labelled B?	
C	In what space (labelled C) is contrast pooling?	
D	Name the structure labelled D.	
E	Name one muscle that inserts into the structure labelled E.	

Case 10.13

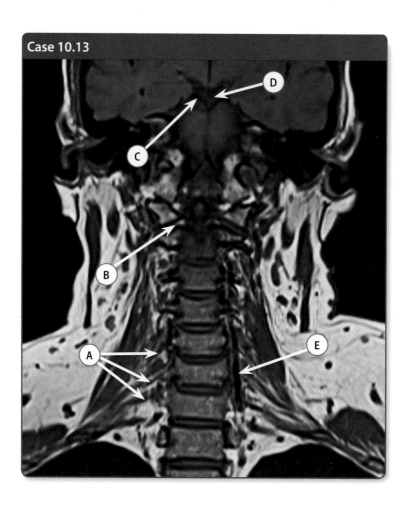

Case 10.13

QUESTION		WRITE YOUR ANSWER HERE
A	Name the structure labelled A.	
B	Name the structure labelled B.	
C	Name the structure labelled C.	
D	Name the structure labelled D.	
E	Name the structure labelled E.	

Case 10.14

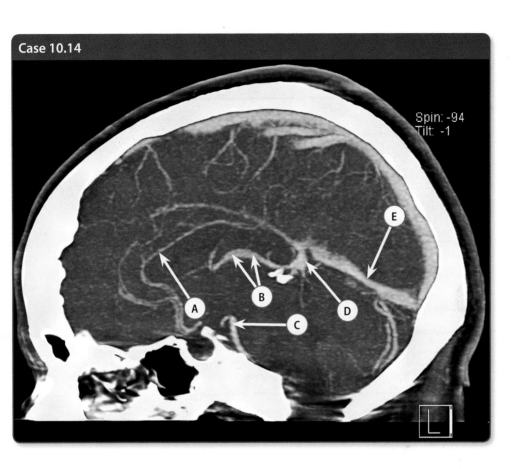

Case 10.14

QUESTION		WRITE YOUR ANSWER HERE
A	Name the structure labelled A.	
B	Name the structure labelled B.	
C	Name the structure labelled C.	
D	Name the structure labelled D.	
E	Name the structure labelled E.	

Case 10.15

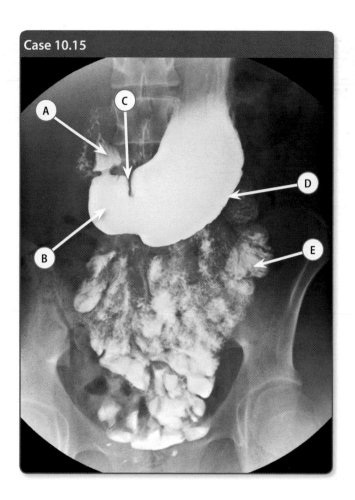

Case 10.15

QUESTION		WRITE YOUR ANSWER HERE
A	Name the structure labelled A.	
B	Name the structure labelled B.	
C	Name the structure labelled C.	
D	Name the structure labelled D.	
E	Name the structure labelled E.	

Case 10.16

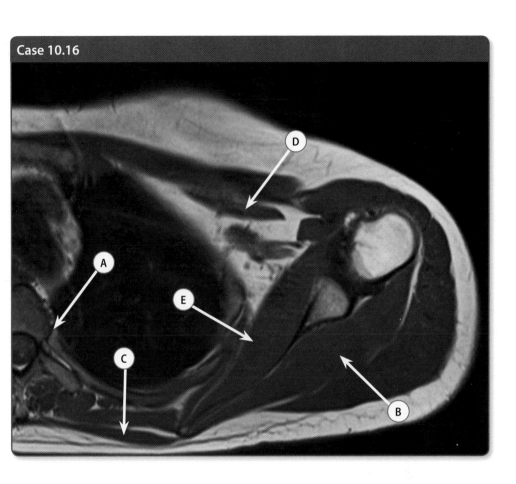

Case 10.16

	QUESTION	WRITE YOUR ANSWER HERE
A	Name the structure labelled A.	
B	Name the structure labelled B.	
C	Name the structure labelled C.	
D	Name the insertion site of the structure labelled D.	
E	Name the structure labelled E.	

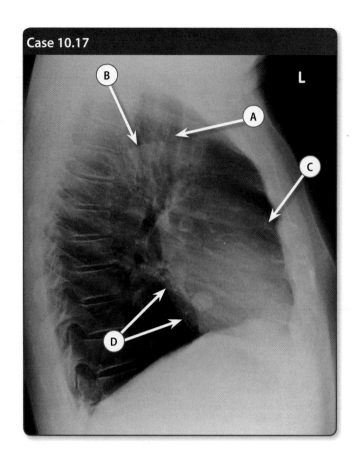

Case 10.17

	QUESTION	WRITE YOUR ANSWER HERE
A	Name the radiolucent structure labelled A.	
B	Name the structure labelled B.	
C	Which chamber of the heart lies anteriorly (C)?	
D	Which chamber of the heart lies posteriorly (D)?	
E	At what level does the trachea usually divide?	

Case 10.18

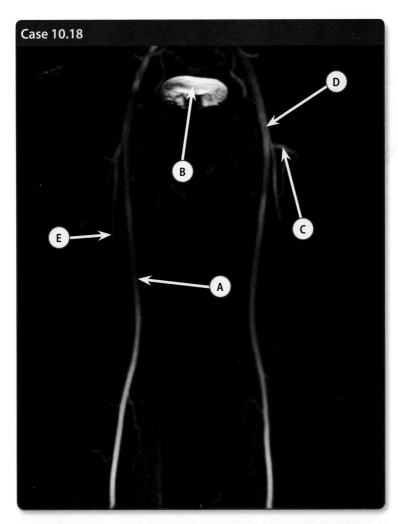

Case 10.18

	QUESTION	WRITE YOUR ANSWER HERE
A	Name the structure labelled A.	
B	Name the structure labelled B.	
C	Name the structure labelled C.	
D	Name the structure labelled D.	
E	Name the structure labelled E.	

Case 10.19

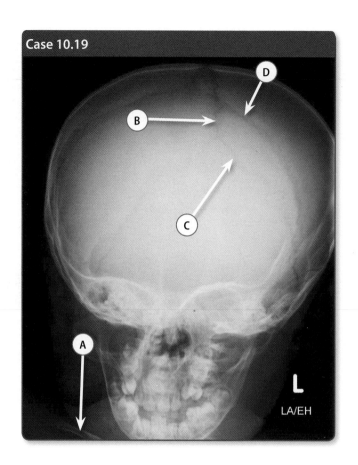

L
LA/EH

Case 10.19

QUESTION		WRITE YOUR ANSWER HERE
A	Name the structure labelled A.	
B	Name the structure labelled B.	
C	Name the structure labelled C.	
D	Name the structure labelled D.	
E	What is the point at which suture B meets suture D (along with its contralateral counterpart) called?	

Case 10.20

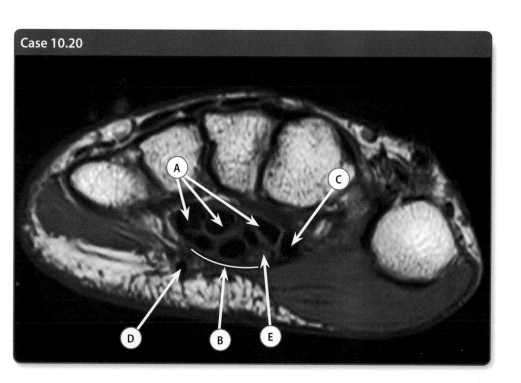

Case 10.20

QUESTION		WRITE YOUR ANSWER HERE
A	Name the structure labelled A.	
B	Name the structure labelled B.	
C	Name the structure labelled C.	
D	Name the structure labelled D.	
E	Name the structure labelled E.	

Answers

Case 10.1

A Right costotransverse joint

B Right transverse process of C6

C Left uncinate process of C5

D Left clavicle

E Left cervical rib

The uncinate process forms the uncovertebral joint (or neurocentral joint of Luschka) with the vertebral body above. Each rib articulates with its thoracic vertebra at two joints: the costotransverse joint, between the tubercle of the rib and the transverse process; and the costovertebral joint, between the head of the rib and articular facets of the vertebral body. Cervical ribs articulate with the C7 vertebra, usually unilaterally, and are present in around 0.2% of the population.

Case 10.2

A Gastric wall

B Portal vein (portal venous confluence)

C Aorta

D Left adrenal gland

E Inferior vena cava

The thickness of the gastric wall on CT examinations is very variable and it is better not to comment on abnormal 'thickness' unless the stomach has been deliberately distended by the patient drinking sufficient fluid. The splenic vein lies immediately posterior to the head, neck and body of the pancreas – without intravenous contrast, differentiation between the two is often impossible. At this level, you will often see areas of altered attenuation within the inferior vena cava (IVC) due to different veins in this vicinity containing varying levels of contrast. These flow artefacts should not be misinterpreted as thrombus.

Case 10.3

A. Lateral tibial plateau (condyle)

B. Posterior horn of lateral meniscus

C. Quadriceps tendon

D. Articular cartilage of lateral femoral condyle

E. Head of fibula

Orientating sagittal images of the knee can be difficult. However, the key clue on this image is the visualisation of the head of fibula, which lies lateral to the tibia.

Being aware of this finding will enable the rest to fall into place:

1.   visualised meniscus = lateral meniscus
2.   tibia = lateral tibial condyle
3.   femur = lateral femoral condyle

(D) is something of a trick question and is reliant on your understanding of MR signal in the region of articulations. Remember, fatty marrow will return high T1-weighted signal, the cortex will return no T1-weighted signal (black) and the cartilage lining the articular surface will return intermediate signal intensity.

Case 10.4

A Left pulmonary artery

B Left superior pulmonary vein

C Left inferior pulmonary vein

D Left atrium

E Four

A delayed angiographic run of a pulmonary arteriogram is used to visualise the pulmonary veins.

There are four pulmonary veins, with a superior and inferior pulmonary vein on each side. There are a number of possible anomalies, including having three pulmonary veins on the right (upper, middle and lower lobes) and fusion of the two veins on the left resulting in a common trunk.

Case 10.5

A Right iliacus muscle

B Intervertebral disc

C Uterus (fundus)

D Left obturator externus muscle

E Right ovary

A doughnut-shaped fundus of the uterus is seen in the coronal plane. Note the appearance of the endometrium, the innermost histological layer of the uterus. It is under hormonal control and undergoes cyclic regeneration. The ovaries are visualised on either side of the uterus, showing characteristic high T2-weighted signal within the ovarian follicles.

Case 10.6

A Right maxillary antrum

B Mandibular division (V3) of the left trigeminal nerve (CN V)

C Left foramen spinosum

D Clivus

E Right external auditory canal

The sphenoid bone contains two major foramina: foramen ovale and foramen spinosum.

- **Foramen ovale** – larger than foramen spinosum. It lies medial to foramen spinosum and transmits the mandibular division of the trigeminal nerve along with the accessory meningeal artery
- **Foramen spinosum** – situated posterolateral to the foramen ovale and transmits the middle meningeal artery and vein

Case 10.7

A Head of pancreas

B Neck of pancreas

C Splenic vein

D Abdominal aorta

E Portal venous confluence

The pancreas is a retroperitoneal structure, and as such is often obscured by bowel gas on ultrasound imaging. The pancreas itself is composed of a head (lying to the right of the midline, with the uncinate process lying inferiorly), neck (which passes the midline anterior to the L1/L2 vertebrae), body and tail (both of which lie to the left of the midline). The confluence of the portal vein is seen to the right of the midline, posteromedial to the head of the pancreas, as it is formed from the splenic vein and the superior mesenteric vein. The abdominal aorta is an indirect posterior relation of the pancreas.

Case 10.8

A Capitulum of distal humerus

B Common flexor tendon

C Coronoid process of ulna

D Proximal diaphysis of radius

E Trochlea of distal humerus

The distal humerus comprises medial and lateral epicondyles, capitulum and trochlea.

The medial epicondyle is the origin for the common flexor tendon, a tendinous origin for the following muscles:

- Pronator teres, flexor carpi radialis, palmaris longus, flexor carpi ulnaris, flexor digitorum superficialis muscles.

The lateral epicondyle is the origin of the common extensor tendon, a tendinous origin for the following muscles:

- Extensor carpi radialis brevis, extensor digitorum, extensor digiti minimi, extensor carpi ulnaris muscles.

Case 10.9

A. Left superior vena cava (SVC)

B. Descending thoracic aorta

C. Oesophagus

D. Trachea

E. Sternum

A persistent left SVC is an anatomical variant which usually drains via the coronary sinus into the right atrium. This occurs due to failure of regression of the left anterior and common cardinal veins and the left sinus horn.

Persistence of the embryonic cardinal vein on the left in addition to a normal vein on the right leads to formation of a double SVC. The right SVC drains into the right atrium and the left into the coronary sinus.

In 10% of individuals with a left SVC, the SVC drains into the left atrium producing an asymptomatic right-to-left shunt. This is commonly present in heterotaxy syndromes.

Case 10.10

A. Superior mesenteric artery (SMA)

B. Jejunal branch of the SMA

C. Middle colic artery

D. Right colic artery

E. Ileocolic artery

The SMA arises from the aorta at the level of L1, approximately 1 cm inferior to the coeliac axis. It travels anteroinferiorly, posterior to the pancreas, and to the left of the superior mesenteric vein. The branches of the SMA include:

1. middle colic artery – supplies the transverse colon
2. right colic artery – supplies the ascending colon
3. ileocolic artery – supplies the ileum, caecum and appendix
4. jejunal branches – supply the jejunum

Case 10.11

A Temporal horn of the right lateral ventricle

B Right hippocampus

C Right lentiform nucleus

D Head of the left caudate nucleus

E Left parahippocampal gyrus

Coronal images nicely depict the medial temporal lobe, especially the hippocampus and parahippocampal gyrus, which are parts of the limbic system. The hippocampus is the area of grey matter which lies adjacent to the temporal horn of the lateral ventricle, forming part of its floor. The parahippocampal gyrus forms the medial aspect of the temporal lobe.

Case 10.12

A Left sacroiliac joint

B Hub of needle

C Joint capsule of the left hip

D Left superior pubic ramus

E Left gluteus minimus, gluteus medius, piriformis, obturator internus or gemellus (superior or inferior) muscles

Fluoroscopic hip arthrography has been replaced by MR arthrography in modern day imaging. However, contrast joint injection is still performed under fluoroscopic guidance and the patient is subsequently imaged using MRI.

When injecting contrast into the joint, it is vital to appreciate the location of the contrast being administered. A puncture overlying the medial femoral head may result in filling of the extra-articular iliopsoas bursa. A successful intra-articular injection will show free flow of contrast around the entirety of the femoral head.

Case 10.13

A. Nerves of the right brachial plexus

B. Right atlanto-axial joint

C. Right posterior cerebral artery

D. Interpeduncular cistern

E. Left vertebral artery

The brachial plexus is formed from the anterior rami of the C5–T1 spinal nerve roots. The components of the brachial plexus have a constant relationship with specific anatomical landmarks, which are easily identifiable on MRI. These include:

- scalene muscles
- atlanto-occipital joint
- cervical portion of the vertebral artery

Case 10.14

  A Pericallosal artery

  B Internal cerebral veins

  C Basilar artery

  D Great vein of Galen

  E Straight sinus

Paired internal cerebral veins join together in the quadrigeminal cistern along with the basal vein of Rosenthal to form the great vein of Galen (great cerebral vein). This is a short single midline vessel which lies under the splenium of the corpus callosum and drains into the straight sinus.

The inferior sagittal sinus lies in the free edge of the falx cerebri.

Case 10.15

  A Duodenal cap

  B Antrum of stomach

  C Incisura angularis

  D Greater curvature of stomach

  E Jejunum

The incisura angularis – or angular notch – lies between the body of the stomach and the antrum. The duodenal cap represents the first part of the duodenum and is intraperitoneal. The duodenum distal to this is retroperitoneal – an important consideration given the difference in radiographic appearances between intraperitoneal and retroperitoneal visceral perforations. The fourth part of the duodenum is continuous with the jejunum at the duodenojejunal flexure.

Case 10.16

  A Left costovertebral joint

  B Left infraspinatus muscle

  C Left trapezius muscle

  D Left coracoid process

  E Left subscapularis muscle

There are two posterior articulations between the ribs and vertebrae:

1. costovertebral joint (A)
2. costotransverse joint

Pectoralis minor inserts into the coracoid process of the scapula, which also serves as the origin for the short head of biceps brachii and coracobrachialis.

The dorsal fossae of the scapula are the sites of origin for the supra- and infraspinatus whilst the ventral subscapular fossa serves as the origin for the subscapularis.

Case 10.17

A Trachea

B Aortic arch

C Right ventricle

D Left atrium

E T4

If not specified, most lateral radiographs will be performed in the left lateral position. There are three important 'retro' spaces:

1. Retrosternal – the heart is usually in contact with the lower third of the sternum. In emphysema, this space may be widened. It may be obliterated in right ventricular hypertrophy.
2. Retrotracheal – posterior to the trachea, anterior to the spine and superior to the aortic arch. Mediastinal adenopathy can opacify this space.
3. Retrocardiac – usually lucent, although basal consolidation or a pleural effusion may obliterate this space.

Case 10.18

A Right superficial femoral artery (SFA)

B Urinary bladder

C Left lateral circumflex femoral artery

D Left common femoral artery (CFA)

E Right profunda femoris artery (PFA)

The CFA is a direct continuation of the external iliac artery from the level of the inguinal ligament. On average, the CFA is around 4 cm in length before branching into the SFA and PFA (deep femoral artery).

Facts:

- PFA arises laterally from the CFA and then courses posterior to the SFA.
- PFA gives rise to the lateral and medial femoral circumflex arteries.

The SFA ends at the lower third of the thigh, passing through an opening in the adductor magnus muscle (medially) known as the adductor hiatus to become the popliteal artery.

Case 10.19

A Right clavicle

B Sagittal suture

C Left lambdoid suture

D Left coronal suture

E Bregma

The sagittal and lambdoid sutures meet posteriorly at the lambda – accordingly, the point at which the paired parietal bones meet the occipital bone. This corresponds to the site of the posterior fontanelle in the fetus or neonate. The sagittal and coronal sutures meet anteriorly at the bregma, as would the anteriorly placed metopic (or frontal) suture, if present. This is therefore where the paired parietal bones meet the frontal bone and corresponds to the site of the anterior fontanelle. This is an important anatomical landmark in neonatal cranial ultrasound. A wormian bone (usually a normal variant) can be seen in the left coronal suture in this case.

Case 10.20

A Flexor digitorum profundus tendons

B Flexor retinaculum

C Flexor pollicis longus tendon

D Ulnar artery

E Median nerve

The carpal tunnel is a fibro-osseous space situated in the ventral aspect of the wrist. The deep boundary is formed by the volar aspect of the carpal bones and the more superficial boundary is formed by the dense fibrous flexor retinaculum. The carpal tunnel contains:

1. the median nerve – fasciculate appearance
2. four flexor digitorum profundus tendons
3. four flexor digitorum superficialis tendons
4. the flexor pollicis longus tendon

Guyon's canal is a space within the wrist which lies between the pisiform and hamate, through which the ulnar artery and ulnar nerve run to the hand.

Chapter 11

Mock paper 11

20 cases to be answered in 75 minutes

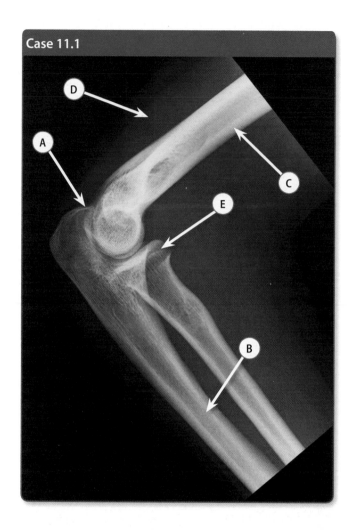

Case 11.1

Case 11.1

QUESTION		WRITE YOUR ANSWER HERE
A	Name the structure labelled A.	
B	Name the structure labelled B.	
C	Name the structure labelled C.	
D	Name the structure labelled D.	
E	Name the structure labelled E.	

Case 11.2

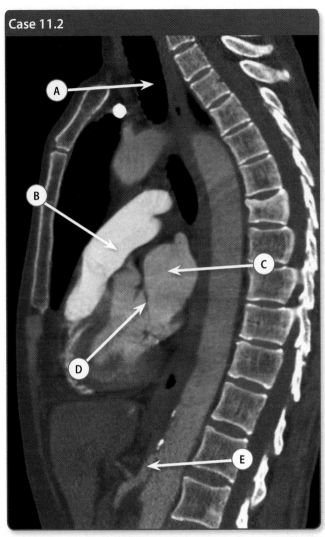

Case 11.2

QUESTION		WRITE YOUR ANSWER HERE
A	Name the structure labelled A.	
B	Name the structure labelled B.	
C	Name the chamber labelled C.	
D	Name the structure labelled D.	
E	Name the structure labelled E.	

Case 11.3

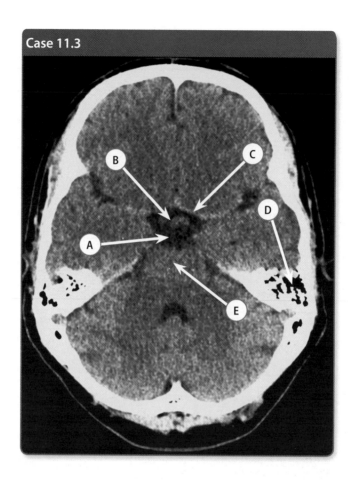

Case 11.3

QUESTION		WRITE YOUR ANSWER HERE
A	Name the structure labelled A.	
B	Name the structure labelled B.	
C	Name the structure labelled C.	
D	Name the structure labelled D.	
E	Name the structure labelled E.	

Case 11.4

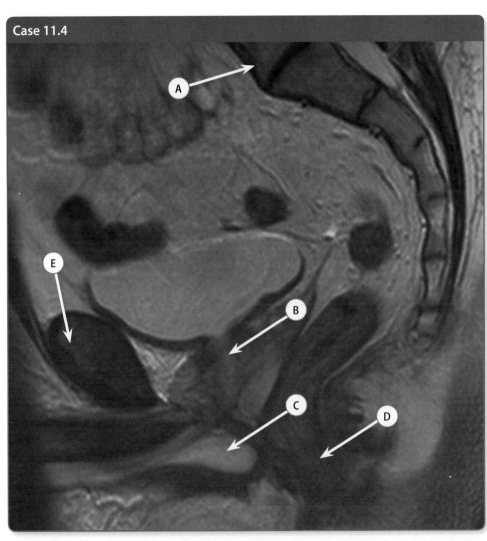

Case 11.4

QUESTION		WRITE YOUR ANSWER HERE
A	Name the structure labelled A.	
B	Name the structure labelled B.	
C	Name the structure labelled C.	
D	Name the structure labelled D.	
E	Name the structure labelled E.	

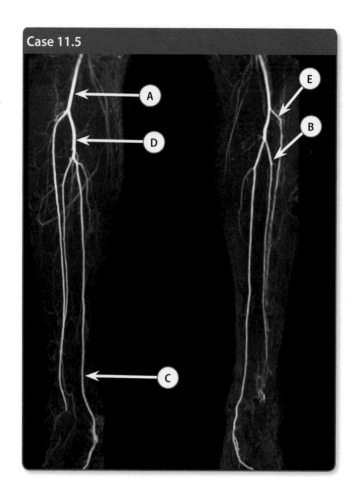

Case 11.5

	QUESTION	WRITE YOUR ANSWER HERE
A	Name the structure labelled A.	
B	Name the structure labelled B.	
C	Where is artery 'C' usually palpable?	
D	Name the structure labelled D.	
E	Name the structure labelled E.	

Case 11.6

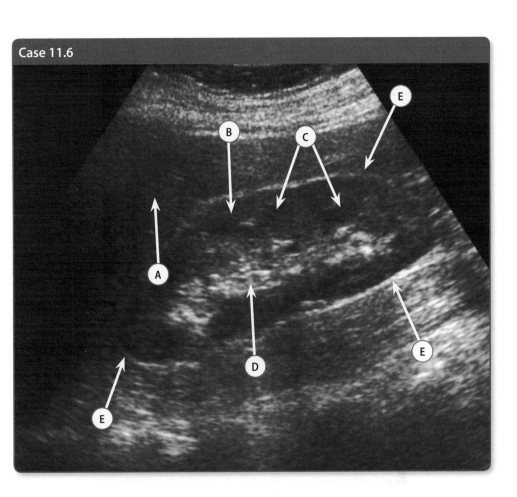

Case 11.6

QUESTION		WRITE YOUR ANSWER HERE
A	Name the structure labelled A.	
B	Name the structure labelled B.	
C	Name the hypoechoic structures labelled C.	
D	Name the echogenic central part of the kidney shown by the letter D?	
E	What is the outer covering of the kidney shown by the letter E?	

Case 11.7

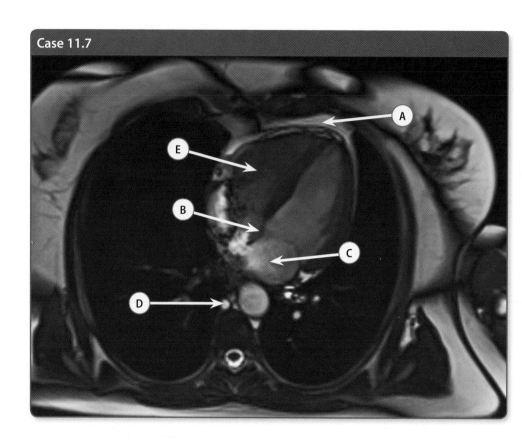

Case 11.7

QUESTION		WRITE YOUR ANSWER HERE
A	Name the structure labelled A.	
B	Name the structure labelled B.	
C	Name the chamber labelled C.	
D	Name the structure labelled D.	
E	Name the structure labelled E.	

Case 11.8

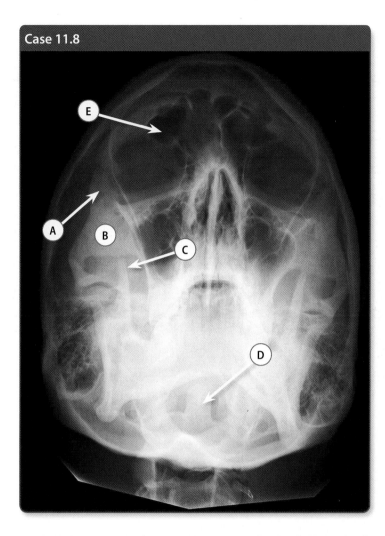

Case 11.8

QUESTION		WRITE YOUR ANSWER HERE
A	Name the structure labelled A.	
B	Name the structure labelled B.	
C	Name the structure labelled C.	
D	Name the structure labelled D.	
E	Name the structure labelled E.	

Case 11.9

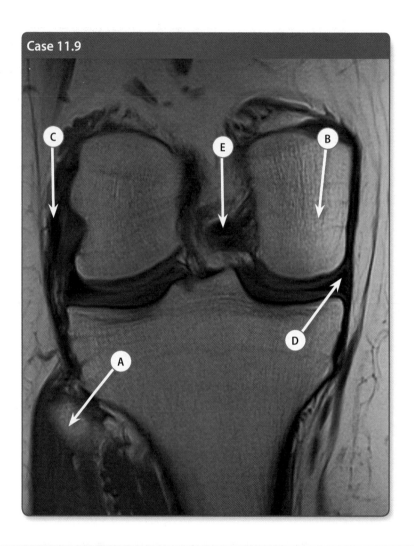

Case 11.9

QUESTION		WRITE YOUR ANSWER HERE
A	Name the structure labelled A.	
B	Name the structure labelled B.	
C	Name the structure labelled C.	
D	Name the structure labelled D.	
E	Name the structure labelled E.	

Case 11.10

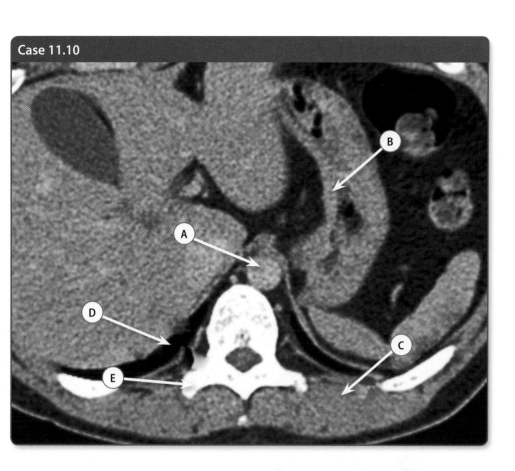

Case 11.10

QUESTION		WRITE YOUR ANSWER HERE
A	Name the structure labelled A.	
B	Name the structure labelled B.	
C	Name the structure labelled C.	
D	Name the structure labelled D.	
E	Name the structure labelled E.	

Case 11.11

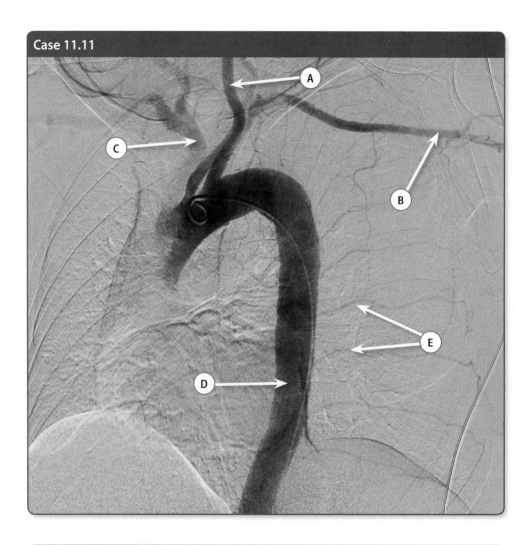

Case 11.11

QUESTION		WRITE YOUR ANSWER HERE
A	Name the structure labelled A.	
B	Name the structure labelled B.	
C	Name the structure labelled C.	
D	Name the structure labelled D.	
E	Name the structure labelled E.	

Case 11.12

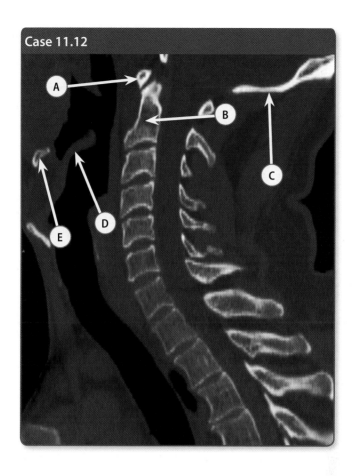

Case 11.12

QUESTION		WRITE YOUR ANSWER HERE
A	Name the structure labelled A.	
B	Name the structure labelled B.	
C	Name the structure labelled C.	
D	Name the structure labelled D.	
E	Name the structure labelled E.	

Case 11.13

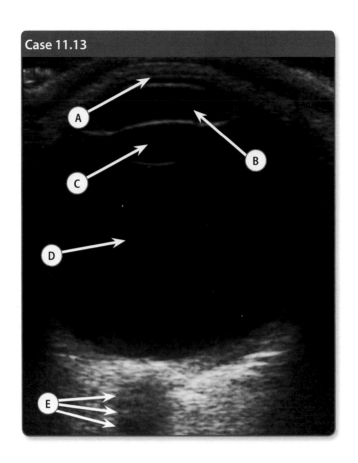

Case 11.13

QUESTION		WRITE YOUR ANSWER HERE
A	Name the structure labelled A.	
B	Name the structure labelled B.	
C	Name the structure labelled C.	
D	Name the structure labelled D.	
E	Name the structure labelled E.	

Case 11.14

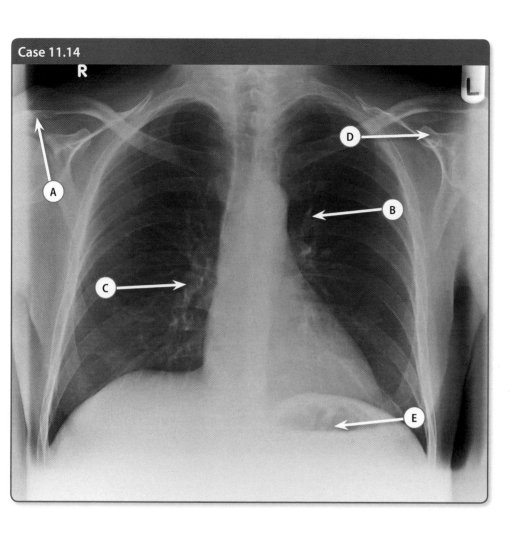

Case 11.14

QUESTION		WRITE YOUR ANSWER HERE
A	Name the joint labelled A.	
B	Name the structure labelled B.	
C	Name the structure labelled C.	
D	Name the structure labelled D.	
E	Name the structure labelled E.	

Case 11.15

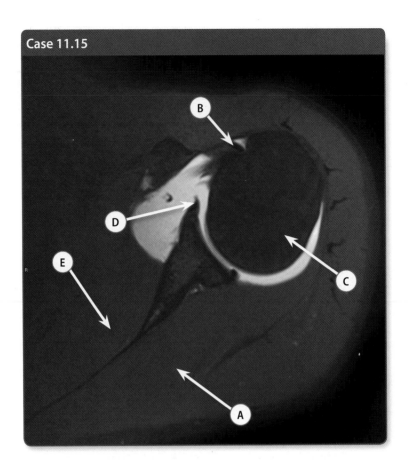

Case 11.15

QUESTION		WRITE YOUR ANSWER HERE
A	Name the structure labelled A.	
B	Name the structure labelled B.	
C	Name the structure labelled C.	
D	Name the structure labelled D.	
E	Name the structure labelled E.	

Case 11.16

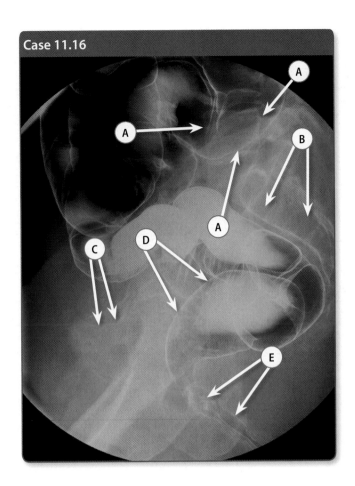

Case 11.16

QUESTION		WRITE YOUR ANSWER HERE
A	Name the osseous structure labelled A.	
B	Name the structure labelled B.	
C	Name the structure labelled C.	
D	Name the structure labelled D.	
E	Name the non-anatomical structure labelled E.	

Case 11.17

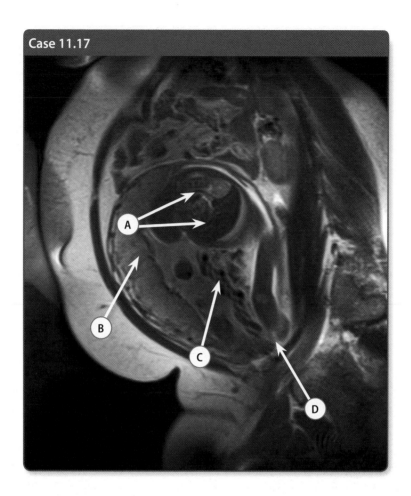

Case 11.17

QUESTION		WRITE YOUR ANSWER HERE
A	Name the structure labelled A.	
B	Name the structure labelled B.	
C	Name the structure labelled C.	
D	Name the structure labelled D.	
E	What are the usual constituent vessels of the umbilical cord?	

Case 11.18

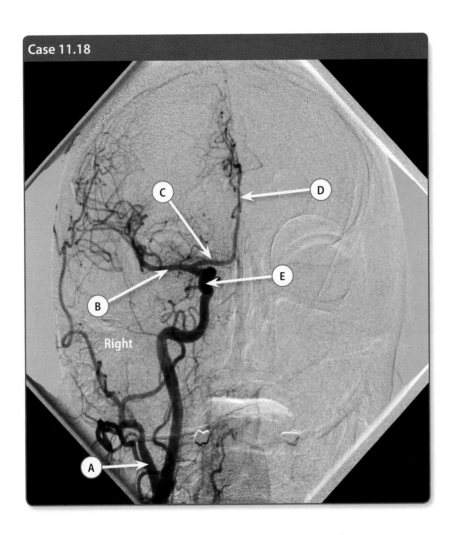

Case 11.18

QUESTION		WRITE YOUR ANSWER HERE
A	Name the structure labelled A.	
B	Name the structure labelled B.	
C	Name the structure labelled C.	
D	Name the structure labelled D.	
E	Name the structure labelled E.	

Case 11.19

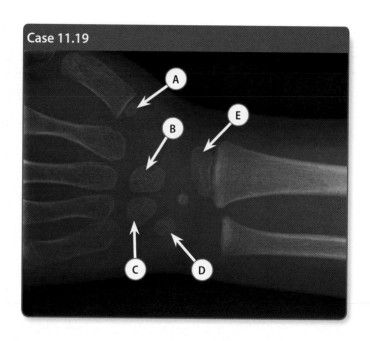

Case 11.19

QUESTION		WRITE YOUR ANSWER HERE
A	Name the structure labelled A.	
B	Name the structure labelled B.	
C	Name the structure labelled C.	
D	Name the structure labelled D.	
E	Name the structure labelled E.	

Case 11.20

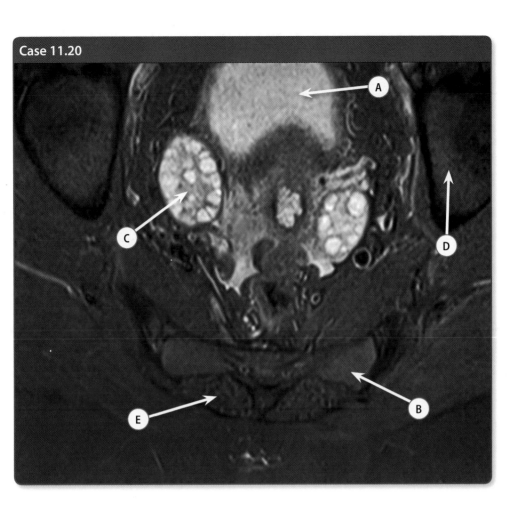

Case 11.20

QUESTION		WRITE YOUR ANSWER HERE
A	Name the structure labelled A.	
B	Name the structure labelled B.	
C	Name the structure labelled C.	
D	Name the structure labelled D.	
E	Name the structure labelled E.	

Answers

Case 11.1

A Olecranon of the ulna

B Proximal diaphysis of the ulna

C Distal diaphysis of the humerus

D Triceps brachii muscle

E Head of radius

On the lateral radiograph of the elbow, the trochlea and capitulum of the distal humerus are superimposed on one another.

There are two fundamental lines that must be reviewed on the lateral radiograph (with the elbow flexed at 90°) in order to confidently exclude displaced fractures and dislocations:

1. The normal anterior humeral line will have at least one third of the capitulum anterior to it. This line is drawn along the anterior aspect of the distal humeral diaphysis and through the elbow joint.
2. The normal radiocapitellar line passes through the middle of the capitulum. This line is drawn centrally through the proximal radius and through the elbow joint.

Case 11.2

A Trachea

B Pulmonary trunk

C Left atrium

D Posterior leaflet of the mitral valve

E Coeliac trunk

The right ventricle is the most anterior chamber of the heart and the pulmonary outflow tracts arises from this. The left atrium is the most posterior chamber and it drains into the left ventricle, with the mitral valve separating the two.

You will also observe that contrast is more dense within the pulmonary arteries than in the aorta and left atrium. This scan is timed to interrogate the pulmonary arteries (CT pulmonary angiogram).

Case 11.3

A Suprasellar cistern

B Optic chiasm

C Left middle cerebral artery

D Left mastoid air cells

E Pons

The shape of the CSF spaces at the level of the suprasellar cistern resembles a 'sad face'. The suprasellar cistern is also described as being star-shaped, as depicted in **Figure 11.1**.

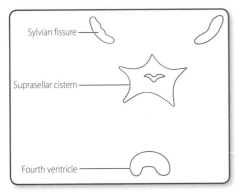

Sylvian fissure

Suprasellar cistern

Fourth ventricle

Figure 11.1 'Sad face.' Schematic illustration of the relationships between CSF spaces at the level of the suprasellar cistern.

Case 11.4

A Body of L5 vertebra

B Prostatic urethra

C Corpus cavernosum

D Rectum

E Symphysis pubis

The male urethra is typically around 20 cm in length. It follows an approximately S-shaped path. From proximal to distal, the named parts are: prostatic, membranous, bulbar and penile.

Case 11.5

A Right popliteal artery

B Left peroneal artery

C Posteroinferior to the medial malleolus

D Right tibioperoneal trunk or right posterior tibial artery

E Left anterior tibial artery

The popliteal artery bifurcates into the anterior and posterior tibial arteries. The posterior tibial artery distal to the origin of the anterior tibial and proximal to the origin of the peroneal artery is also known as the tibioperoneal trunk.

An easy way to remember the three vessel runoff of the lower limb is: **APP** (like Android or Apple apps)

- **A**nterior tibial artery – lateral
- **P**eroneal artery
- **P**osterior tibial artery – medial

The peroneal artery is sandwiched between the anterior tibial and posterior tibial arteries.

Case 11.6

A Right lobe of liver

B Renal cortex

C Renal pyramids

D Renal sinus

E Renal capsule

The right kidney is optimally visualised on ultrasound imaging by using the liver as an acoustic window. The contrasting echogenicity at the interface between the renal capsule and the perirenal fat enables the outline of the kidney to be clearly demonstrated. The renal pyramids are so called because of their shape, with bases lying parallel to the renal capsule and apices pointing towards the renal pelvis. Columns of renal cortex known as the columns of Bertin pass between each renal pyramid. A high fatty content renders the renal sinus very echogenic.

Case 11.7

A Pericardial fat

B Membranous interventricular septum

C Left atrium

D Azygos vein

E Right ventricle

Chambers of the heart are easily identified by their location, with the right system situated more anteriorly and the left system more posteriorly. The membranous portion of the interventricular septum is the more superior thinner portion and is the most common site (80%) of ventricular septal defects. The muscular portion is the greater portion of the septum. Each part has an embryologically distinct origin. The muscular part develops from the bulboventricular flange, which forms as a result of differential growth of primitive ventricle and bulbous cordis. The membranous part has a neural crest origin.

Case 11.8

A Frontal process of right zygoma

B Body of right zygoma

C Coronoid process of right mandible

D Odontoid process (dens) of axis (C2)

E Right frontal sinus

Water's projection is useful for assessing for facial fractures. On this view, the zygoma, orbit and maxilla form the outline of an elephant's head, (**Figure 11.2**). The frontal process of zygoma forms the elephant's forehead, the orbit its ear, the body of zygoma its face and the temporal process of zygoma its trunk.

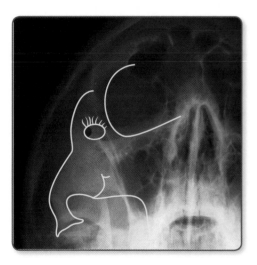

Figure 11.2 'Elephant's head'. A schematic illustration of facial bone relationships on the Water's projection.

Case 11.9

A Head of fibula

B Medial femoral condyle

C Lateral (fibular) collateral ligament

D Medial meniscus

E Posterior cruciate ligament

A useful tool for being able to differentiate between the anterior cruciate ligament (ACL) and the posterior cruciate ligament (PCL) is:

- ACL demonstrates striations
- PCL returns a more uniform low signal and is thicker than the ACL

The head of fibula is (just) visible in this image, thus allowing you to orientate yourself and confidently label (D) as the medial meniscus and (B) as the medial femoral condyle.

The lateral collateral ligament is composed of multiple structures including the biceps femoris tendon, the fibular collateral ligament and the iliotibial band.

Case 11.10

A Aorta

B Lesser curve of stomach

C Left erector spinae muscle

D Lower lobe of the right lung

E Right transverse process of T12

Familiarise yourself with axial views of CTs at various levels. Note the low attenuation gallbladder which lies anterolaterally and is surrounded by liver parenchyma. Views at L1 and L2 are particularly important as an examination favourite for depicting the upper abdominal solid viscera, unpaired aortic branches and upper gastrointestinal tract.

Case 11.11

A Left common carotid artery

B Left axillary artery

C Brachiocephalic trunk/innominate artery

D Descending thoracic aorta

E Left Intercostal vessels

The intercostal arterial branches are evident on this example. There are a total of eleven posterior intercostal arteries on each side. The upper two arise from the superior intercostal artery, which is a branch of the costocervical trunk of the subclavian artery. The lower nine paired branches arise from the thoracic aorta and travel along the inferior border of the corresponding rib. Each artery travels in a neurovascular bundle along with a posterior intercostal vein and intercostal nerve.

The artery is sandwiched between the vein (which lies above) and the nerve (below). Hence, the mnemonic **VAN** can be used to recall the order of the **V**ein, **A**rtery and **N**erve.

Case 11.12

A Anterior arch of C1

B Odontoid peg

C Occipital bone

D Epiglottis

E Body of hyoid bone

The distance between the odontoid peg (dens) and the anterior arch of C1 is known as the atlantodental interval. In the context of trauma, an increase in the atlantodental interval to more than 3 mm in adults or 5 mm in children is suggestive of atlantoaxial subluxation. Sagittal reformats are also useful for examining the alignment of facet joints. Facet joint dislocation may be seen on sagittal views as 'perched' facets.

Case 11.13

A Cornea

B Aqueous humour

C Lens

D Vitreous humour

E Optic sheath

This is an axial ultrasound of the orbit. Dynamic imaging of the eye can be obtained with ultrasound, using the eyelid as an acoustic window. The wall of the ocular globe has a multilayered coat with the most outer layer formed by fibrous sclera, the middle layer by vascular choroid and the inner layer by the very thin retina. Internally, the ocular globe contains structures with high water content, namely aqueous humour, vitreous humour and the lens. These appear hypoechoic on ultrasound.

The optic sheath covers the optic complex (optic nerve and ophthalmic artery); this cannot be readily identified with conventional 2D ultrasound.

Case 11.14

A Right acromioclavicular joint

B Left upper lobe pulmonary vein

C Right lower lobe pulmonary artery

D Left coracoid process of scapula

E Gastric fundus

The hila are composed of major bronchi, blood vessels and lymphatics. The hila may be seen at the same level but commonly, the left is higher than the right because of the position of the left main bronchus, over which the left upper lobe pulmonary artery courses.

The hilar points are the angles formed by the descending upper lobe veins and descending pulmonary arteries. Not every normal patient has a very clear hilar point on both sides, but if present, they can be useful indicators of disease processes.

Case 11.15

   A Infraspinatus muscle

   B Long head of biceps brachii tendon

   C Head of humerus

   D Anterior glenoid labrum

   E Subscapularis muscle

The long head of biceps tendon originates from the supraglenoid tubercle of the scapula and courses down the proximal humerus in the bicipital groove. The subscapularis muscle lies deep to the body of the scapula whereas the infraspinatus muscle lies superficially.

Case 11.16

   A Vertebral body of L5

   B Sacrum

   C Superior pubic ramus

   D Rectum

   E Rectal contrast tube in anal canal

This image shows the rectum and sigmoid colon in double contrast. Haustra are an important means of differentiating large bowel from small bowel radiographically, but are characteristically absent in the rectum. Taeniae coli are three longitudinal muscle bands which are shorter than the overall length of the unstretched colon and as such result in colonic sacculations (and therefore haustra) between the caecum and sigmoid colon. However, these bands merge to form a complete muscle layer around the rectum meaning that haustra are absent.

The presacral space (posterior to the rectum and anterior to the sacrum and coccyx) is an important review area on lateral views on barium enema examinations, with widening of the space raising suspicions for the presence of such pathologies as tumour, meningocoele and abscess.

Case 11.17

   A Fetus

   B Placenta

   C Umbilical cord

   D Uterine cervix

   E Two umbilical arteries, one umbilical vein

Parasagittal MRI acquisition of a pregnant patient and fetus (seen at (A)). The placenta is evident at (B) with its inferior aspect located distant to the cervix in an obstetrically favourable position. The umbilical cord is seen at (C) in a typical spiral pattern. Two umbilical arteries and one vein usually make up the umbilical cord. The umbilical artery joins the internal iliac artery of the fetus and drain deoxygenated blood to the placenta. The single umbilical vein delivers oxygenated blood to the fetus via the ductus venosum. In adulthood the vein regresses to form the falciform ligament.

Case 11.18

A Right external carotid artery

B Right middle cerebral artery

C Right anterior cerebral artery

D Right pericallosal artery

E Cavernous portion of the right internal carotid artery

The intracranial portion of the internal carotid artery (ICA) gives off three major branches:

- **Anterior cerebral artery (ACA)** – a smaller terminal branch which runs anteromedially, close to the midline, on the medial surface of the hemisphere in the interhemispheric fissure. Both ACAs are linked by the anterior communicating artery
- **Middle cerebral artery** – the largest terminal branch which runs inferolaterally through the Sylvian fissure between the frontal and temporal lobes
- **Posterior communicating artery** – runs posteriorly and connects with the ipsilateral posterior cerebral artery, forming the posterior portion of the circle of Willis and connecting anterior and posterior circulations.

Case 11.19

A First metacarpal epiphysis

B Capitate

C Hamate

D Triquetral

E Distal radial epiphysis

The ossification status of the bones of the hand and wrist is used to evaluate skeletal maturity ('bone age'), e.g. in precocious puberty or growth restriction. The capitate and hamate are the first two carpal bones to ossify (within the first year of life) and as such are seen here to be the two most developed carpal bones. The triquetral is usually the next carpal bone to ossify, followed by the lunate (the smallest ossification centre to be seen here). No further carpal ossification centres are evident in this case. The pisiform is typically the last of the carpal bones to ossify.

Case 11.20

A Urinary bladder

B Left sacral alum

C Right ovary

D Left (superior) acetabulum

E Right erector spinae muscle

The osseous acetabulum is composed of a triad of pelvic bones – the pubic bone, ischium and ilium. On careful examination of the image, the low signal of the cortices of the femoral heads is just visible thus allowing (D) to be identified as the superior acetabulum.

This axial oblique image clearly demonstrates the functional follicles in the paired ovaries.

Chapter 12

Mock paper 12

20 cases to be answered in 75 minutes

Case 12.1

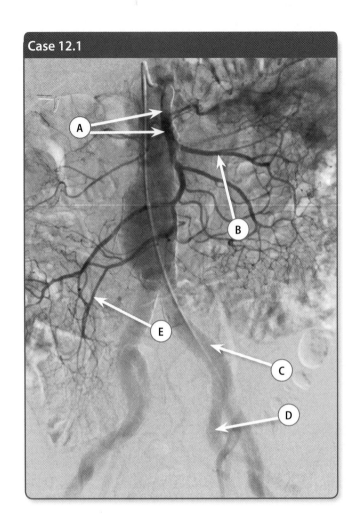

Case 12.1

QUESTION		WRITE YOUR ANSWER HERE
A	Name the structure labelled A.	
B	Name the structure labelled B.	
C	Name the structure labelled C.	
D	Name the structure labelled D.	
E	Name the structure labelled E.	

Case 12.2

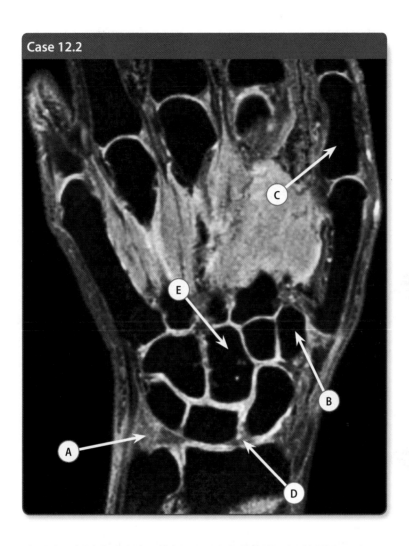

Case 12.2

QUESTION		WRITE YOUR ANSWER HERE
A	Name the structure labelled A.	
B	Name the structure labelled B.	
C	Name the structure labelled C.	
D	Name the structure labelled D.	
E	Name the structure labelled E.	

Case 12.3

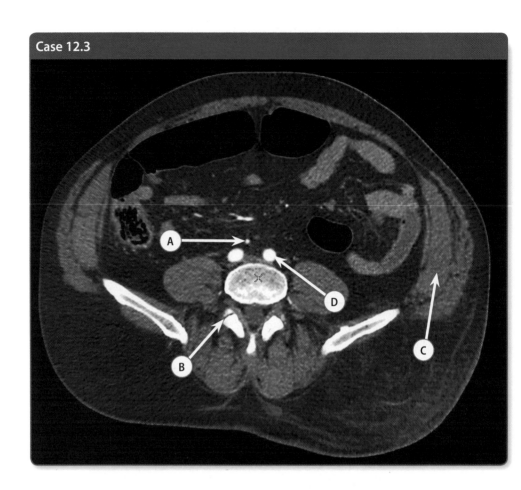

Case 12.3

QUESTION		WRITE YOUR ANSWER HERE
A	Name the structure labelled A.	
B	Name the structure labelled B.	
C	Name the structure labelled C.	
D	Name the structure labelled D.	
E	What is the usual maximum diameter of the common iliac arteries in an adult patient?	

Case 12.4

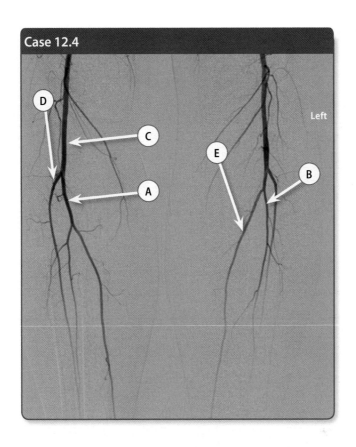

Case 12.4

QUESTION		WRITE YOUR ANSWER HERE
A	Name the structure labelled A.	
B	Name the structure labelled B.	
C	Name the structure labelled C	
D	Name the structure labelled D.	
E	Name the structure labelled E.	

Case 12.5

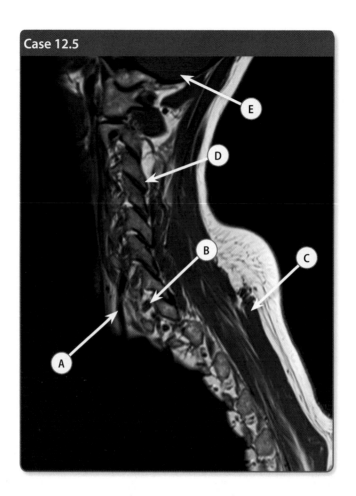

Case 12.5 Left parasagittal T1-weighted MRI of cervical spine	
QUESTION	WRITE YOUR ANSWER HERE
A Name the structure labelled A.	
B What is the nerve root labelled B?	
C Name the structure labelled C.	
D Name the structure labelled D.	
E Name the structure labelled E.	

Case 12.6

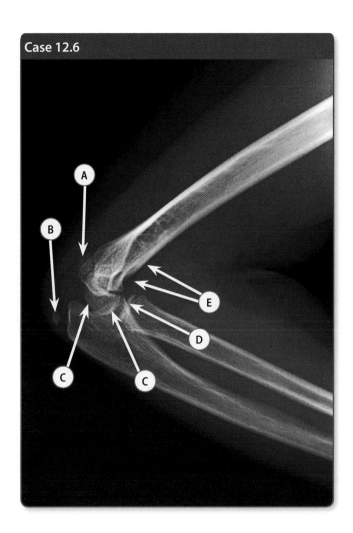

Case 12.6

QUESTION		WRITE YOUR ANSWER HERE
A	Name the structure labelled A.	
B	Name the structure labelled B.	
C	Name the structure labelled C.	
D	Name the structure labelled D.	
E	What does the dark line shown by E correspond to?	

Case 12.7

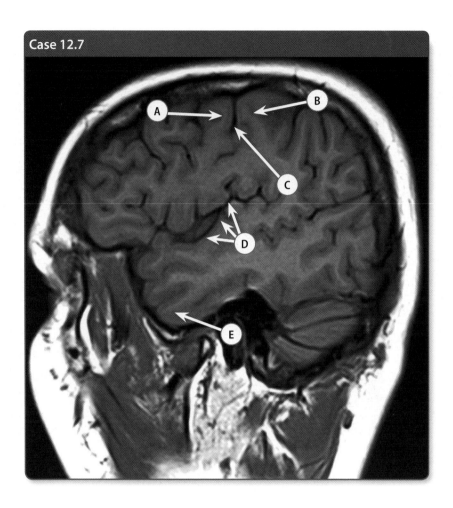

Case 12.7

QUESTION		WRITE YOUR ANSWER HERE
A	Name the structure labelled A.	
B	Name the structure labelled B.	
C	Name the structure labelled C.	
D	Name the structure labelled D.	
E	Name the structure labelled E.	

Case 12.8

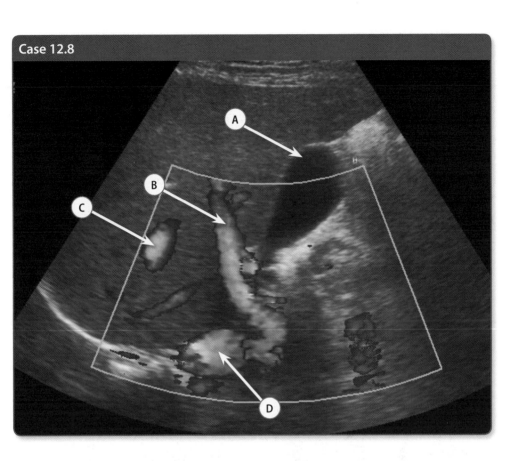

Case 12.8

QUESTION		WRITE YOUR ANSWER HERE
A	Name the structure labelled A.	
B	Name the structure labelled B.	
C	Name the structure labelled C.	
D	Name the structure labelled D.	
E	From what two structures is structure B usually formed?	

Case 12.9

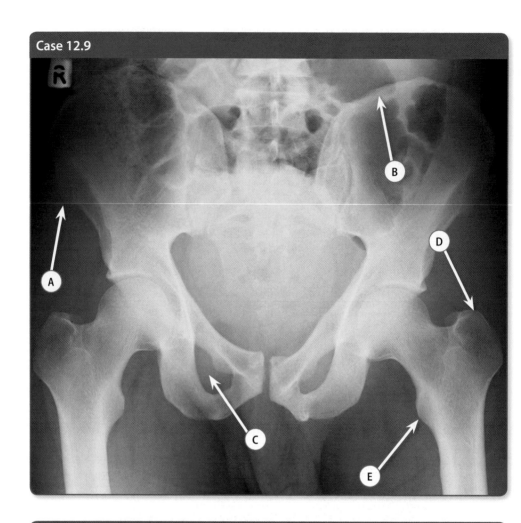

Case 12.9

QUESTION		WRITE YOUR ANSWER HERE
A	What muscle originates from A?	
B	Name the osseous structure labelled B.	
C	What nerve passes through C?	
D	Name one muscle that inserts into the structure labelled D.	
E	What muscle inserts into the structure labelled E?	

Case 12.10

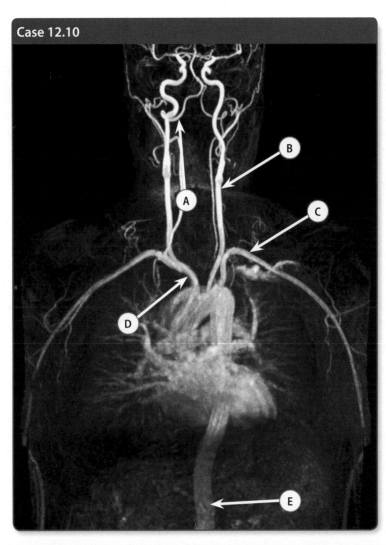

Case 12.10

QUESTION		WRITE YOUR ANSWER HERE
A	Name the structure labelled A.	
B	Name the structure labelled B.	
C	Name the structure labelled C.	
D	Name the structure labelled D.	
E	Name the structure labelled E.	

Case 12.11

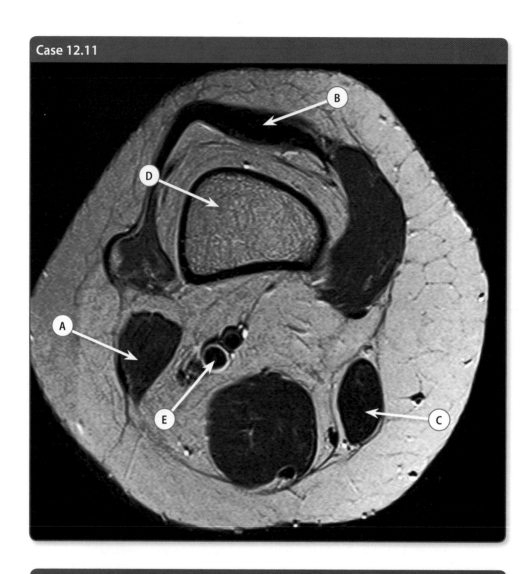

Case 12.11

QUESTION		WRITE YOUR ANSWER HERE
A	Name the structure labelled A.	
B	Name the structure labelled B.	
C	Name the structure labelled C.	
D	Name the structure labelled D.	
E	Name the structure labelled E.	

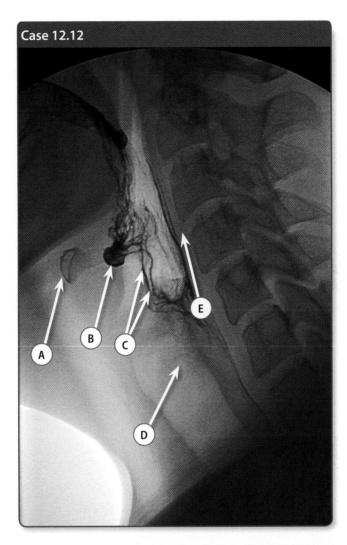

Case 12.12

QUESTION		WRITE YOUR ANSWER HERE
A	Name the structure labelled A.	
B	Name the structure labelled B.	
C	Name the structure labelled C.	
D	Name the structure labelled D.	
E	Name the structure labelled E.	

Case 12.13

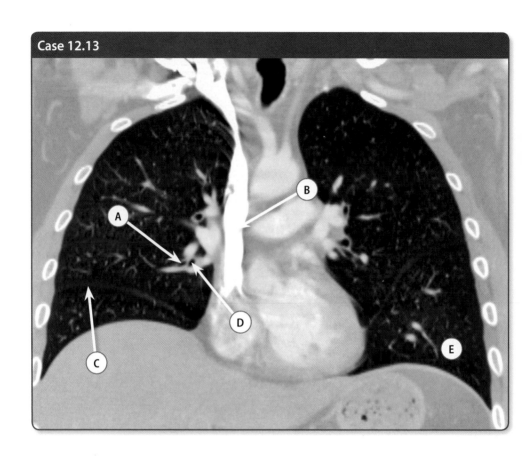

Case 12.13

QUESTION		WRITE YOUR ANSWER HERE
A	Name the structure labelled A.	
B	Name the structure labelled B.	
C	Name the structure labelled C.	
D	Name the structure labelled D.	
E	What bronchopulmonary segment is labelled E?	

Case 12.14

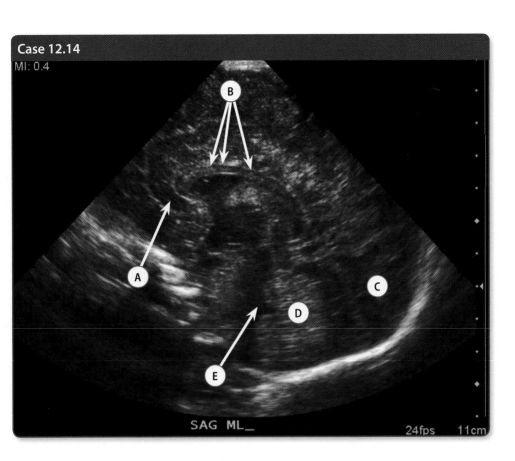

Case 12.14

QUESTION		WRITE YOUR ANSWER HERE
A	Name the structure labelled A.	
B	Name the structure labelled B.	
C	Name the structure labelled C.	
D	Name the structure labelled D.	
E	Name the structure labelled E.	

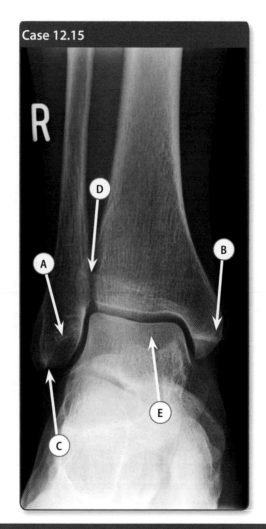

Case 12.15

Case 12.15		
QUESTION		**WRITE YOUR ANSWER HERE**
A	Name the structure labelled A.	
B	Name the structure labelled B.	
C	Name a tendon that passes via the space labelled C.	
D	Name the structure labelled D.	
E	Name the structure labelled E.	

Case 12.16

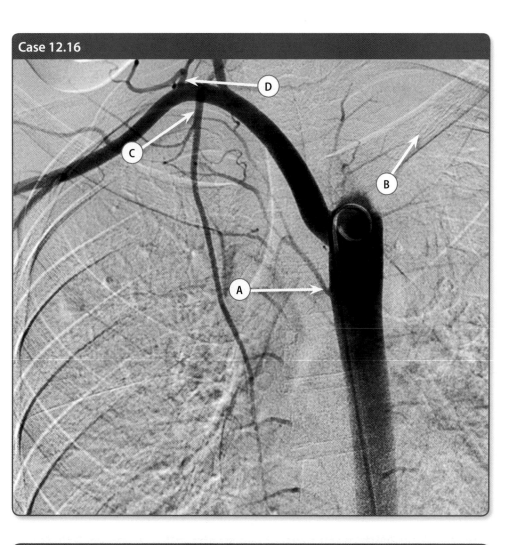

Case 12.16

QUESTION		WRITE YOUR ANSWER HERE
A	Name the structure labelled A.	
B	Name the structure labelled B.	
C	Name the structure labelled C.	
D	Name the structure labelled D.	
E	Which anatomical variant is present on this image?	

Case 12.17

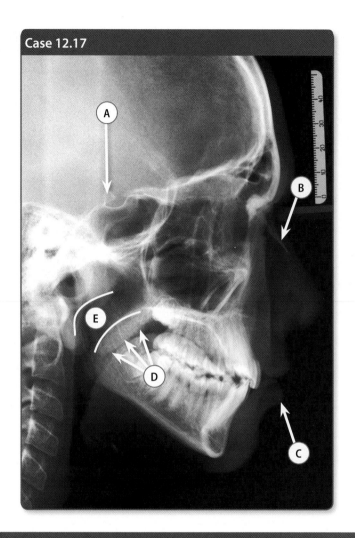

Case 12.17

QUESTION		WRITE YOUR ANSWER HERE
A	Name the structure labelled A.	
B	Name the structure labelled B.	
C	Name the structure labelled C.	
D	Name the structure labelled D.	
E	Name the space E lying between the two lines.	

Case 12.18

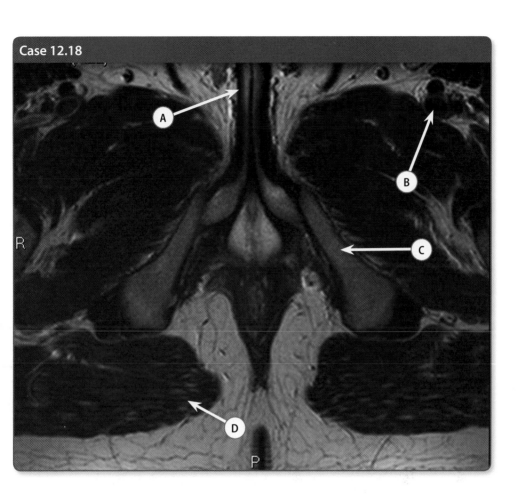

Case 12.18

QUESTION		WRITE YOUR ANSWER HERE
A	Name the structure labelled A.	
B	Name the structure labelled B.	
C	Name the structure labelled C.	
D	Name the structure labelled D.	
E	Name the non-paired erectile column of the penis.	

Case 12.19

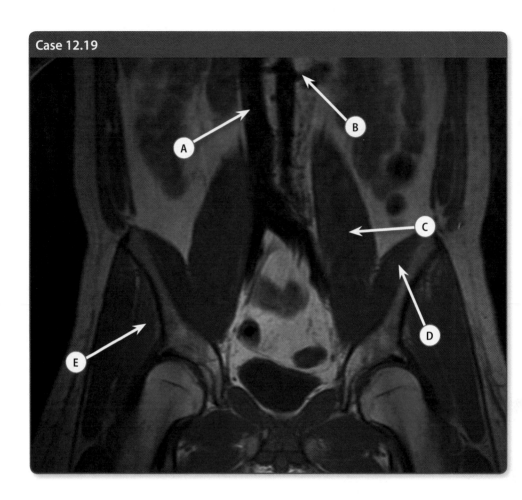

Case 12.19

QUESTION		WRITE YOUR ANSWER HERE
A	Name the structure labelled A.	
B	Name the structure labelled B.	
C	Name the structure labelled C.	
D	Name the structure labelled D.	
E	Name the structure labelled E.	

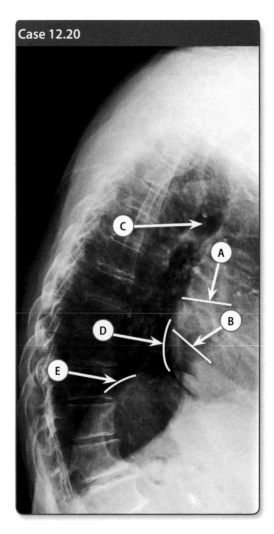

Case 12.20

Case 12.20

QUESTION		WRITE YOUR ANSWER HERE
A	Name the linear structure labelled A.	
B	Name the linear structure labelled B.	
C	Name the lucent structure labelled C.	
D	Name the cardiac chamber outlined by label D.	
E	Name the linear structure labelled E.	

Answers

Case 12.1

A Superior mesenteric artery (SMA)

B Branches to jejunum

C Left common iliac artery

D Left internal iliac artery

E Ileocolic branch of SMA

The SMA supplies the small bowel and the proximal large bowel up to the mid transverse colon.

If you are a James Bond fan, you may find the following phrase useful for memorising the SMA branches: Sean Connery In froM Russia wIth Love:

- Inferior pancreaticoduodenal
- Middle colic
- Right colic
- Intestinal
- iLeocolic

Case 12.2

A Triangular fibrocartilage complex

B Trapezium

C Proximal phalanx of the thumb

D Scapholunate ligament

E Capitate

Mnemonic for the carpal bones:

Scared Lovers Try Positions That They Cannot Handle

Proximal carpal row (from radial to ulnar)
Scaphoid, Lunate, Triquetral, Pisiform

Distal carpal row (from radial to ulnar)
Trapezium, Trapezoid, Capitate, Hamate

Remember – trapeziUM is by the thUMb (the thUMb swings on the trapeziUM).

Case 12.3

A Inferior mesenteric artery (IMA)

B Right facet joint

C Left internal oblique muscle

D Left common iliac artery

E 2 cm

The IMA is seen anterior to the common iliac arteries. The IMA arises from the anterior aorta at the level of L3 and supplies the colon from the distal transverse colon to the rectum. Major branches include the left colic artery, sigmoid artery and superior rectal branches.

Case 12.4

A Right tibioperoneal trunk (posterior tibial artery)

B Left peroneal artery

C Right popliteal artery

D Right anterior tibial artery

E Left posterior tibial artery

A mnemonic for the distal three vessel runoff in the lower limb is **APP**:

1. **A**nterior tibial artery – most superior branch (lateral – remember, **AT** is l**AT**eral)

2. **P**eroneal artery – sandwiched in the middle

3. **P**osterior tibial artery – most medial branch.

Another useful tool to help remember which artery branches off first is the use of alphabetical order.

- A comes before **P** – anterior tibial artery being the first branch
- E comes before **O** – p**E**roneal artery is sandwiched between the anterior tibial and p**O**sterior tibial arteries.

Case 12.5

A Left vertebral artery

B Exiting left T1 nerve root

C Left trapezius muscle

D Left inferior articular process of C4

E Left cerebellar hemisphere

The vertebral artery is seen here coursing superiorly after arising from the left subclavian artery. It passes through the foramina transversaria of C6 upwards before forming the basilar artery with its contralateral counterpart. The nerve root seen here exits below the left pedicle of T1 and accordingly will be the left T1 nerve root. The nerve root above this pedicle is the C8 nerve root, and more superiorly in the cervical spine the nerve root exits above its correspondingly numbered pedicle. The superior and inferior articular processes are clearly seen to articulate at the facet joints on this image.

Case 12.6

A Medial epicondyle ossification centre

B Olecranon ossification centre

C Capitulum ossification centre

D Radial head ossification centre

E Anterior fat pad

The anterior fat pad corresponds to the intracapsular layer of fat located between the synovial membrane and the capsular ligament in the coronoid fossa – this is a normal finding. However, in the context of trauma, elevation of this fat pad, or visualisation of a posterior fat pad (i.e. intracapsular fat between the synovial membrane and capsular ligament in the olecranon fossa) is strongly suggestive of an elbow joint effusion and implies the presence of a fracture. The olecranon ossification centre (usually the penultimate ossification centre to be visualised, with the lateral epicondyle representing the last ossification centre to develop) is best appreciated on the lateral view. The medial epicondyle ossification centre should normally overlap the posterior aspect of the humerus on the lateral view; if not, avulsion should be suspected.

Case 12.7

A Precentral gyrus

B Postcentral gyrus

C Central sulcus (Rolandic fissure)

D Lateral sulcus (Sylvian fissure)

E Inferior temporal gyrus

Cerebral hemispheres are divided into lobes by fissures. Each lobe is further subdivided into gyri by sulci. The most constant cortical sulci are as follows:

- **Central sulcus (Rolandic fissure)** – runs coronally and separates the frontal and parietal lobes
- **Parieto-occipital fissure** – divides parietal and occipital lobes
- **Temporo-occipital incisure** – marks the division between temporal and occipital lobes
- **Lateral sulcus (Sylvian fissure)** – separates temporal and parietal lobes

It is also useful to be able to recognise the most constant cortical gyri:

- Pre- and post-central gyri – lie on each side of the central sulcus
- Superior, middle and inferior temporal gyri
- Superior, middle and inferior frontal gyri

Case 12.8

A Gallbladder

B Portal vein

C Middle hepatic vein

D Inferior vena cava (IVC)

E Splenic vein and superior mesenteric vein

The portal vein is usually formed by the superior mesenteric vein and splenic vein (which itself usually receives the inferior mesenteric vein). The portal vein, along with the hepatic artery (shown on this image as the circle lying between the portal vein and the neck of the gallbladder), represents the blood supply to the liver. In the normal physiological state, the portal vein exhibits hepatopetal flow, i.e. flow of blood towards the liver. The hepatic veins, of which there are usually three (right, middle and left) converge on the IVC, joining it just below the inferior cavoatrial junction.

Case 12.9

A Right rectus femoris muscle

B Left iliac crest

C Right obturator nerve

D Left gluteus medius or minimus muscle

E Left iliopsoas muscle

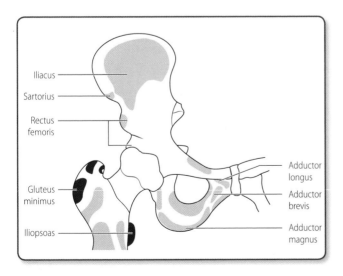

Figure 12.1 Selected muscle origins and insertions of the pelvis.

Case 12.10

A Right vertebral artery

B Left common carotid artery

C Left subclavian artery

D Brachiocephalic trunk/innominate artery

E Abdominal aorta

This MR angiogram shows the normal arterial anatomy of the mediastinum and neck. The brachiocephalic trunk gives rise to the right subclavian artery and right common carotid artery, with the left common carotid artery and left subclavian artery representing the next two branches of the aortic arch in most individuals.

Case 12.11

A Biceps femoris muscle

B Quadriceps tendon

C Sartorius muscle

D Femur

E Popliteal vein

Quadriceps femoris is subdivided into four heads comprising: rectus femoris (superficially); vastus intermedius; vastus lateralis; and vastus medialis (all deep). All four muscles have a conjoined attachment to the patella via the quadriceps tendon.

The popliteal artery and vein lie within the floor of the popliteal fossa with the vein being more superficial – an easy way to remember this is from ultrasound scans for suspected deep venous thrombosis, in which the more superficial vein is compressible in normal patients.

Case 12.12

A Body of the hyoid bone

B Vallecula

C Piriform fossae

D Trachea

E Retropharyngeal soft tissues

The **hypopharynx** is the most inferior part of the pharynx, extending from the inferior margin of the valleculae to the oesophagus (level of C6 vertebrae).

The **piriform fossa** (from the Latin for 'pear-shaped') is the lateral recess of the hypopharynx at the laryngeal orifice.

The **vallecula** (from the Latin for 'valley') is a depression on the anterior hypopharyngeal wall, anterior to the epiglottis. It serves as a landmark dividing the oropharynx and hypopharynx.

Case 12.13

A Lateral segmental bronchus of middle lobe

B Superior vena cava

C Right oblique fissure

D Medial segmental bronchus of middle lobe

E Lateral basal segment of left lower lobe

The right lung comprises three lobes: the upper lobe, middle lobe and lower lobe. There is no middle lobe in the left lung, although the lingula of the left upper lobe serves as its homologue. The middle lobe consists of lateral and medial bronchopulmonary segments. Consolidation in the middle lobe will result in loss of clarity (loss of silhouette) of the right heart border.

Case 12.14

A Cingulate gyrus

B Body of corpus callosum

C Occipital lobe

D Cerebellum

E Fourth ventricle

Cranial ultrasound in a neonate is a safe diagnostic tool. The midline plane is a standard view which gives a good overview of the appearances of the gross anatomy of the supra- and infratentorial brain.

Although it is unlikely to be an investigation you will encounter in everyday clinical practice, approach it by applying basic sonographic rules (fluid is black and soft tissues are grey) and with knowledge of the anatomical structures seen on the midsagittal MRI of the brain, with which with you may be more familiar.

Case 12.15

A Right lateral malleolus

B Right medial malleolus

C Right peroneal brevis/longus tendons

D Right distal tibiofibular syndesmosis

E Dome of the right talus

Structural stability of the ankle is provided by numerous bone and ligamentous articulations, most notably involving the distal tibia and fibula. The distal tibiofibular syndesmosis acts as a fulcrum of stability of the ankle joint which, if disrupted, renders any ankle injury unstable.

The medial malleolus is a pyramidal process of the distal tibia. The lateral malleolus is the terminal fibula. The malleoli provide horizontal stability of the joint due to their strong ligamentous attachments.

The medial flexors of the ankle, which run under the medial malleolus, include: Tom, Dick and Harry – **T**ibialis posterior, flexor **D**igitorum longus, and flexor **H**allucis longus.

The lateral flexors of the ankle, the tendons of which run under the lateral malleolus, include peroneus brevis and peroneus longus.

Case 12.16

A Right costo-bronchial trunk

B Left clavicle

C Right internal mammary artery

D Right costocervical trunk

E Aberrant right subclavian artery

An aberrant right subclavian artery is seen arising directly from the aortic arch. Branches of the subclavian artery are seen to arise as normal. This variant is important when considering vascular intervention.

Case 12.17

A Posterior clinoid process

B Nasal bone

C Lower lip

D Soft palate

E Nasopharynx

Lateral views of the facial bones are taken for two main reasons: for cephalometric measurements in dentistry prior to orthodontic treatment; and in paediatric radiology for assessment of upper airways patency.

It is important to be able to recognise the soft tissue structures visible on the plain radiograph, outlined by air in the upper respiratory tract, such as the soft palate, prevertebral soft tissues and the tongue. The air-filled parts of the aerodigestive tract are also clearly demonstrated, including the oral and nasal cavities, paranasal sinuses, oropharynx, nasopharynx and larynx.

Case 12.18

A Right corpus cavernosum

B Left femoral vein

C Left inferior pubic ramus

D Right gluteus maximus muscle

E Corpus spongiosum

The two corpora cavernosa are seen anteriorly. Posteriorly, they expand bilaterally into the crura of the penis with the ischiocavernous muscles lying immediately adjacent to the bulb of the penis, anterior to the anus, on the internal aspect of the inferior pubic rami. Posterior to these structures lie the fat-filled ischioanal fossae.

Case 12.19

A Inferior vena cava

B Left renal artery

C Left psoas major muscle

D Left iliacus muscle

E Right gluteus minimus muscle

On MRI, flowing blood is depicted as dark flow voids, as seen here in the aorta and inferior vena cava (IVC). The normal configuration of aorta and IVC is shown with the aorta lying to the left of the IVC. The embryology of the IVC is complicated and congenital variations are relatively common (for example, double IVCs or absent sections at varying levels).

Case 12.20

A Horizontal fissure

B Oblique fissure

C Trachea

D Posterior wall of the left atrium

E Left hemidiaphragm

The oblique fissure usually begins at the T4/5 level and runs anteriorly to pass through the hilum. The left oblique fissure is steeper than the right.

The right horizontal fissure runs from the hilum anteriorly at about the level of the fourth rib.

The left hemidiaphragm appears to be higher than the right on the current radiograph but this is projectional as the fundal gas shadow is seen beneath it.

Chapter 13

Mock paper 13

20 cases to be answered in 75 minutes

Case 13.1

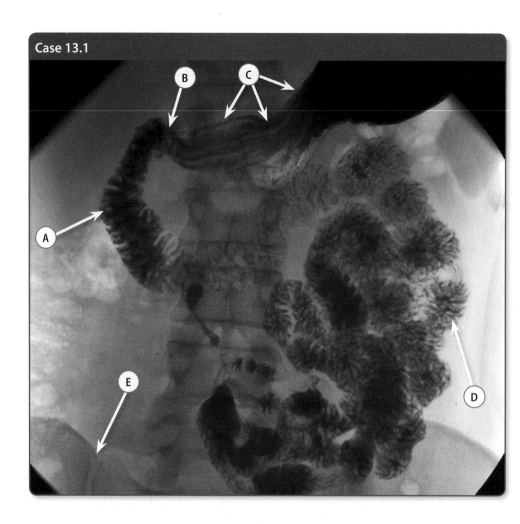

Case 13.1

QUESTION		WRITE YOUR ANSWER HERE
A	Name the structure labelled A.	
B	Name the structure labelled B.	
C	Name the structure labelled C.	
D	Name the structure labelled D.	
E	Name the structure labelled E.	

Case 13.2

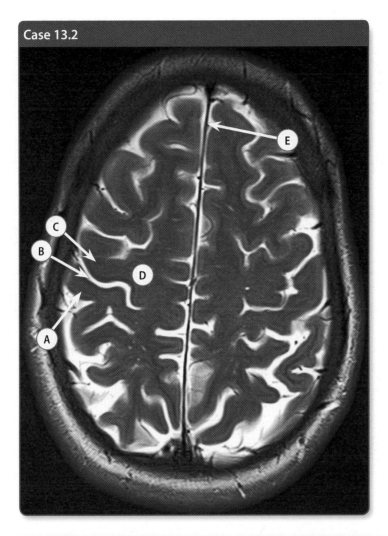

Case 13.2

QUESTION		WRITE YOUR ANSWER HERE
A	Name the structure labelled A.	
B	Name the structure labelled B.	
C	Name the structure labelled C.	
D	Name the structure labelled D.	
E	Name the structure labelled E.	

Case 13.3

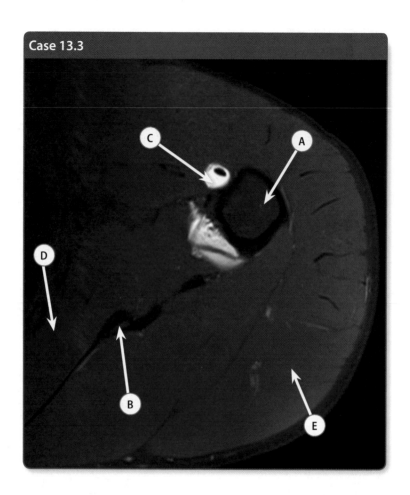

Case 13.3

QUESTION		WRITE YOUR ANSWER HERE
A	Name the structure labelled A.	
B	Name the structure labelled B.	
C	In what space is the contrast labelled C found?	
D	Name the structure labelled D.	
E	Name the structure labelled E.	

Case 13.4

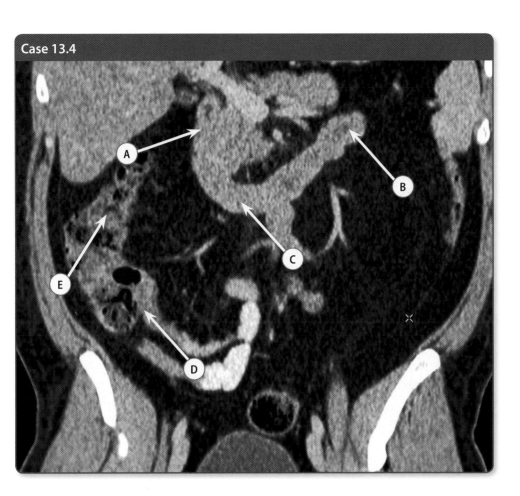

Case 13.4

QUESTION		WRITE YOUR ANSWER HERE
A	Name the structure labelled A.	
B	Name the structure labelled B.	
C	Name the structure labelled C.	
D	Name the structure labelled D.	
E	Name the structure labelled E.	

Case 13.5

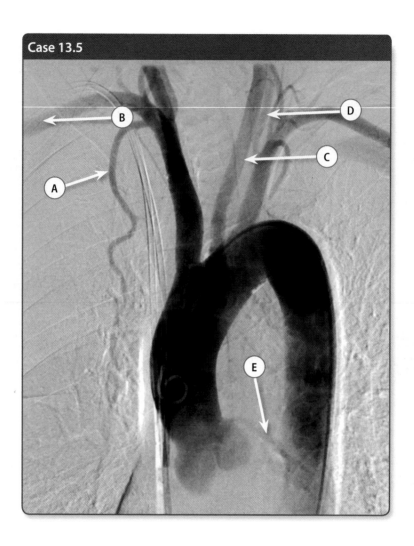

Case 13.5

QUESTION		WRITE YOUR ANSWER HERE
A	Name the structure labelled A.	
B	Name the structure labelled B.	
C	Name the structure labelled C.	
D	Name the structure labelled D.	
E	Name the structure labelled E.	

Case 13.6

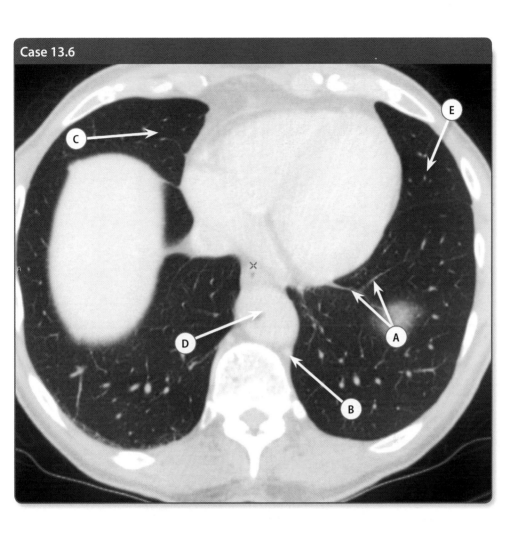

Case 13.6

QUESTION		WRITE YOUR ANSWER HERE
A	What anatomical variant is marked A?	
B	Name the structure labelled B	
C	Which segment of the lung is labelled C?	
D	Name the structure labelled D.	
E	Which segment of the lung is labelled E?	

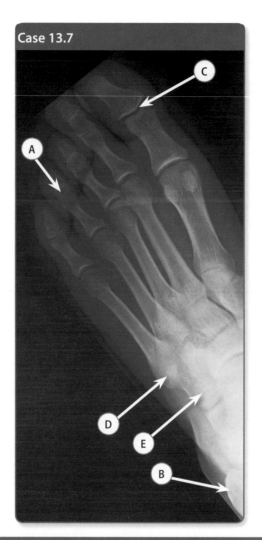

Case 13.7

Case 13.7

QUESTION		WRITE YOUR ANSWER HERE
A	Name the structure labelled A.	
B	Name the structure labelled B.	
C	Name the structure labelled C.	
D	Name the tendon which attaches to the structure labelled D.	
E	Name the structure labelled E.	

Case 13.8

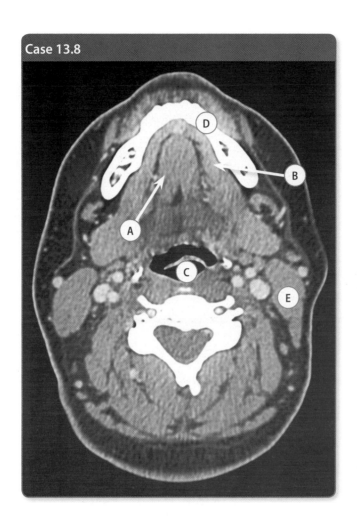

Case 13.8

QUESTION		WRITE YOUR ANSWER HERE
A	Name the structure labelled A.	
B	Name the structure labelled B.	
C	Name the structure labelled C.	
D	Name the structure labelled D.	
E	Name the structure labelled E.	

Case 13.9

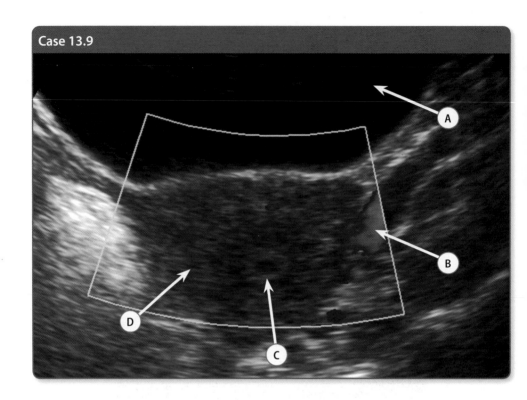

Case 13.9

QUESTION		WRITE YOUR ANSWER HERE
A	Name the structure labelled A.	
B	Name the structure labelled B.	
C	Name the structure labelled C.	
D	Name the structure labelled D.	
E	From which artery does the right uterine artery normally arise?	

Case 13.10

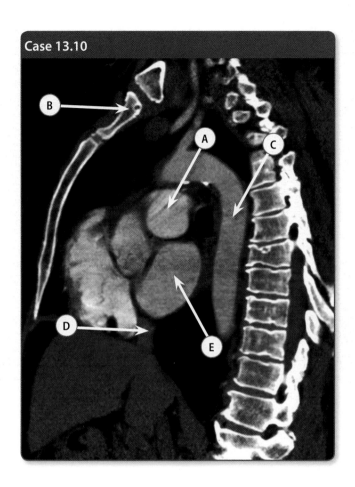

Case 13.10

QUESTION		WRITE YOUR ANSWER HERE
A	Name the structure labelled A.	
B	Name the structure labelled B.	
C	Name the structure labelled C.	
D	Name the structure labelled D.	
E	Name the chamber labelled E.	

Case 13.11

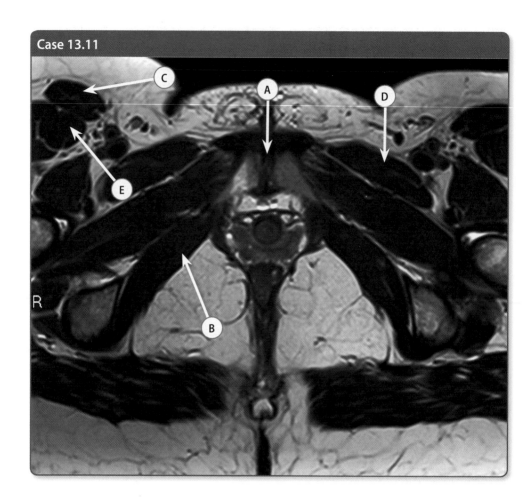

Case 13.11

QUESTION		WRITE YOUR ANSWER HERE
A	Name the structure labelled A.	
B	Name the structure labelled B.	
C	Name the structure labelled C.	
D	Name the structure labelled D.	
E	Name the structure labelled E.	

Case 13.12

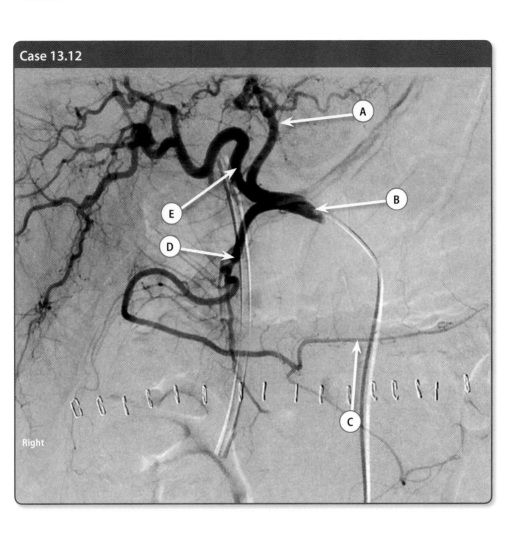

Right

Case 13.12

QUESTION		WRITE YOUR ANSWER HERE
A	Name the structure labelled A.	
B	Name the structure labelled B.	
C	Name the structure labelled C.	
D	Name the structure labelled D.	
E	Name the structure labelled E.	

Case 13.13

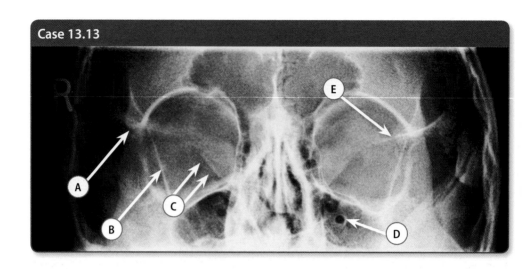

Case 13.13

QUESTION		WRITE YOUR ANSWER HERE
A	Name the suture labelled A.	
B	Name the structure labelled B.	
C	Name the lucent structure labelled C.	
D	Name the structure labelled D.	
E	Name the structure labelled E.	

Case 13.14

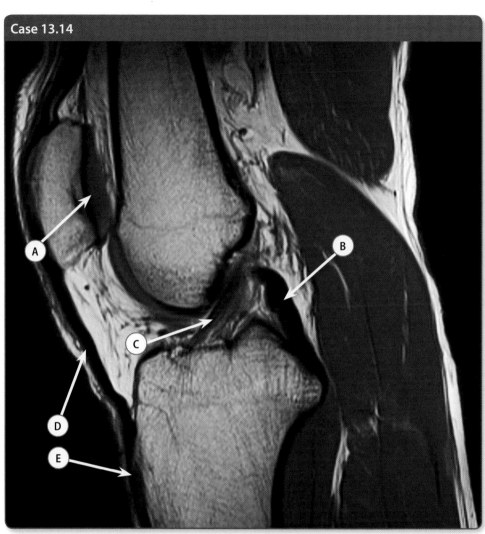

Case 13.14

QUESTION		WRITE YOUR ANSWER HERE
A	Name the structure labelled A.	
B	Name the structure labelled B.	
C	Name the structure labelled C.	
D	Name the structure labelled D.	
E	Name the structure labelled E.	

Case 13.15

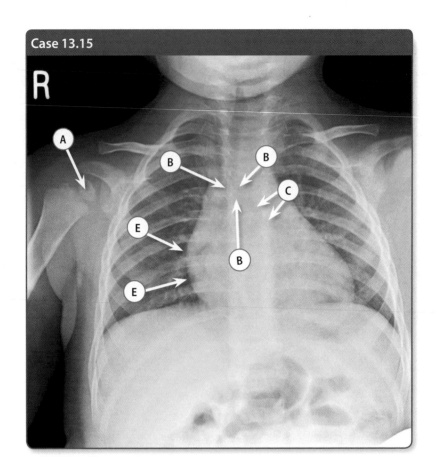

Case 13.15

QUESTION		WRITE YOUR ANSWER HERE
A	Name the structure labelled A.	
B	Name the part of the airways tract labelled B.	
C	Name the part of the airways tract labelled C.	
D	Name the most posterior cardiac chamber.	
E	Name the cardiac chamber that forms the right heart border.	

Case 13.16

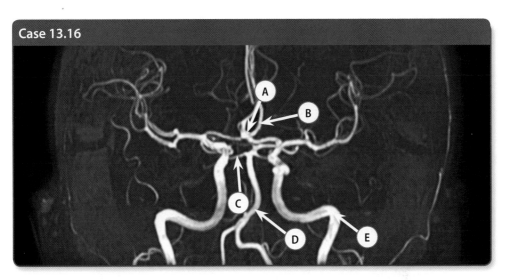

Case 13.16

QUESTION		WRITE YOUR ANSWER HERE
A	Name the structure labelled A.	
B	Name the structure labelled B.	
C	Name the structure labelled C.	
D	Name the structure labelled D.	
E	Name the structure labelled E.	

Case 13.17

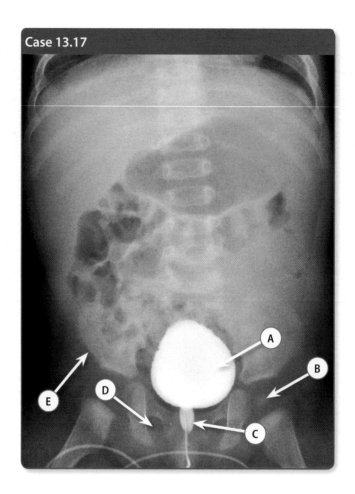

Case 13.17

	QUESTION	WRITE YOUR ANSWER HERE
A	Name the structure labelled A.	
B	Name the structure labelled B.	
C	Name the structure labelled C.	
D	Name the structure labelled D.	
E	Name the osseous structure labelled E.	

Case 13.18

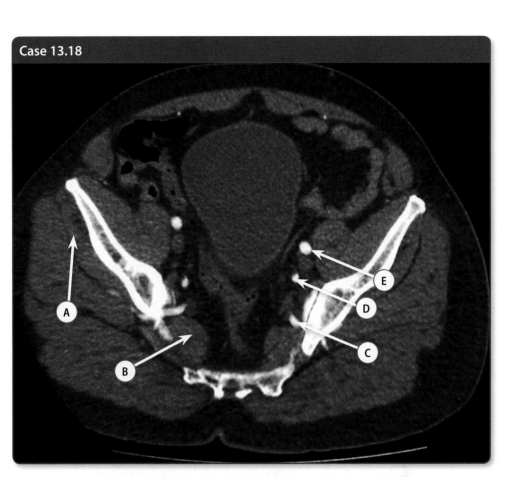

Case 13.18

QUESTION	WRITE YOUR ANSWER HERE
A Name the structure labelled A.	
B Name the structure labelled B.	
C Name the structure labelled C.	
D Name the structure labelled D.	
E Name the structure labelled E.	

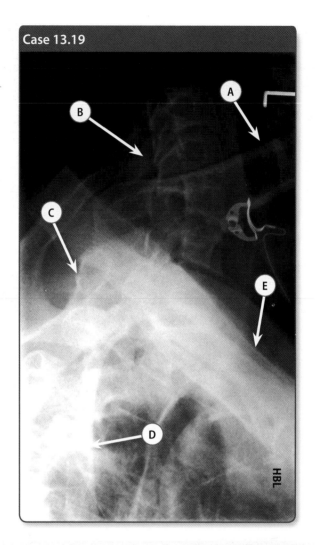

Case 13.19

	QUESTION	WRITE YOUR ANSWER HERE
A	Name the structure labelled A.	
B	Name the structure labelled B.	
C	Name the structure labelled C.	
D	Name the structure labelled D.	
E	Name the structure labelled E.	

Case 13.20

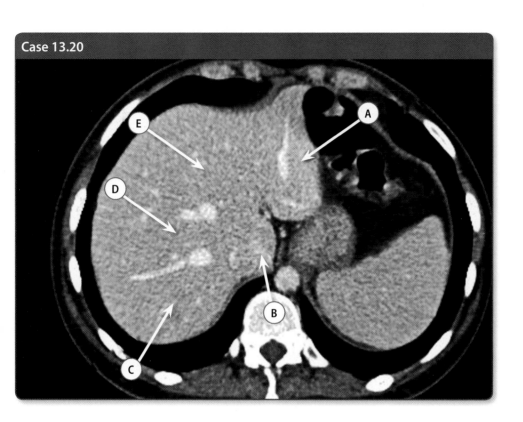

Case 13.20

QUESTION		WRITE YOUR ANSWER HERE
A	Name the liver segment labelled A.	
B	Name the liver segment labelled B.	
C	Name the liver segment labelled C.	
D	Name the liver segment labelled D.	
E	Name the liver segment labelled E.	

Answers

Case 13.1

   A Duodenum (second part)

   B Pylorus

   C Lesser curve of the stomach

   D Jejunum

   E Right sacroiliac joint

The distal stomach, duodenum and proximal small bowel are visualised on this contrast examination.

The stomach consists of body, fundus, cardia and pylorus. It has a more superior lesser curvature and an inferior greater curvature. Try to be specific with recognised gastric nomenclature when answering questions relating to the stomach.

Case 13.2

   A Right postcentral gyrus

   B Right central sulcus (of Rolando)

   C Right precentral gyrus

   D Centrum semiovale

   E Interhemispheric fissure/falx cerebri

The motor pathways travel from the precentral gyrus of the cerebral cortex, via the motor nuclei of the brainstem, to the spinal cord. There are three intracranial portions of the motor pathways:

- **Centrum semiovale** – from the cortex to the roof of the lateral ventricles
- **Corona radiata** – medial part, extending from the level of the roof of the lateral ventricles to the internal capsule
- **Internal capsule** – V-shaped area between the caudate and lentiform nuclei in the basal ganglia

Case 13.3

   A Proximal humerus

   B Body of scapula

   C Long head of biceps brachii tendon sheath

   D Subscapularis muscle

   E Deltoid muscle

The long head of biceps brachii originates from the supraglenoid tubercle (as a tendon) and is enclosed by a sheath which is continuous with the glenohumeral joint – hence contrast is visualised within the sheath outlining the (black) tendon. The tendon lies within the bicipital groove of the most proximal humerus, which is an osseous sulcus created by the lesser and greater tuberosities of the humerus.

Deltoid is seen to lie superficial to the rotator cuff and inferior to the horizontal margin of the clavicle. Trapezius is superior to the clavicle.

Subscapularis originates from the subscapular fossa on the deep/ventral surface of the scapula.

Case 13.4

A Second part of duodenum

B Fourth part of duodenum

C Third part of duodenum

D Ileocecal junction (valve)

E Ascending colon

The duodenum is the proximal part of the small bowel. For descriptive purposes it is divided into four parts, which in the coronal plane form an approximate 'C' shape, as illustrated on this image. The second (descending) part is the location of the ampulla, through which the biliary tree drains into the duodenal lumen. Only the first part of the duodenum is intraperitoneal, with the rest of the duodenum lying in the retroperitoneum. Blood supply to the duodenum is from branches of the coeliac axis and superior mesenteric artery (superior and inferior pancreaticoduodenal arteries respectively).

Case 13.5

A Right internal mammary/thoracic artery

B Right subclavian artery

C Left common carotid artery

D Left vertebral artery

E Left coronary artery

This is a DSA angiogram of the aortic arch, left anterior oblique (LAO) projection. LAO is the best projection to view the unfolded aortic arch. A number of anatomical variants may arise here and it is important to look out for these, particularly when considering vascular intervention.

Common variations to look out for include:

1. Aberrant right subclavian artery arising distal to the origin of the left subclavian artery
2. Common origin of the left common carotid artery and the brachiocephalic trunk

Case 13.6

  A Left inferior accessory fissures

  B Hemiazygos vein

  C Medial segment of the middle lobe

  D Descending thoracic aorta

  E Inferior segment of the lingula

Accessory fissures are seen on up to 10% of chest radiographs and 20% of CT scans. The inferior accessory fissures separate the medial and the lateral basal segments of the lower lobes. They can be easily mistaken for linear atelectasis or pleural bands.

On the current slice, the oblique fissures can be seen at both lung bases. On the right, it separates the middle lobe (abutting the heart) from the lower lobe. On the left, it separates the left upper lobe from the lower lobe.

Case 13.7

  A Middle phalanx of fourth toe

  B Lateral malleolus/distal fibula

  C Interphalangeal joint of great toe

  D Peroneus brevis tendon

  E Cuboid

The fundamentals will allow you to score full marks for this question:

1. The great toe only has two phalanges, hence interphalangeal joint
2. The base of the fifth metatarsal is the insertion site for the peroneal brevis tendon, one of the two lateral ankle flexors
3. The cuboidal bone articulates with the bases of the fourth and fifth metatarsals
4. The medial, intermediate and lateral cuneiforms articulate with the first, second and third metatarsal bases respectively.

Case 13.8

  A Right genioglossus muscle

  B Left mylohyoid muscle

  C Oropharynx

  D Body of the mandible

  E Left sternocleidomastoid muscle

The floor of the mouth is the inferior boundary of the oral cavity, lying beneath the tongue. The floor of the mouth is divided by the mylohyoid muscle (which forms the oral diaphragm) into two spaces:

- Sublingual – superomedial
- Submandibular – inferolateral

Two other important muscles that help form the floor of the mouth are genioglossus and the anterior belly of digastric.

Case 13.9

A Urinary bladder

B Left external iliac vessels

C Endometrium

D Body of uterus/myometrium

E Anterior division of right internal iliac artery

The urinary bladder should be full for transabdominal ultrasound imaging of the female pelvis to enable satisfactory visualisation of the pelvic viscera. The most central hypoechoic area in the uterus represents fluid within the uterine cavity. The hyperechoic ring around this is the endometrium, the thickness of which depends on the stage of the menstrual cycle in premenopausal women. A hypoechoic ring around the endometrium corresponds to the innermost layer of myometrium. The uterine arteries are tortuous vessels which arise from the anterior divisions of the internal iliac arteries – an anatomical fact that is important when considering endovascular intervention of uterine fibroids or in obstetric haemorrhage.

Case 13.10

A Pulmonary trunk

B Manubrium of sternum

C Descending thoracic aorta

D Inferior vena cava

E Left atrium

The main pulmonary trunk is identified within the concavity of the aortic arch. The aortopulmonary window (the fat-containing space between the aortic arch and the pulmonary artery) is also noted. The ligamentum arteriosum and the left recurrent laryngeal nerve lie within this window.

The left atrium is the most posterior cardiac chamber and is thus a useful anatomical landmark when assessing cross-sectional images.

Case 13.11

A Symphysis pubis

B Right obturator internus muscle

C Right sartorius muscle

D Left pectineus muscle

E Right rectus femoris muscle

The symphysis pubis is a cartilaginous midline joint formed between the pubic bones. The pubic bones serve as an origin of multiple muscles, including:

• pectineus
• adductor magnus (shared origin)
• adductor longus
• adductor brevis
• gracilis

Another important landmark for the muscle origins includes the ischial tuberosity of the ischium. It provides the origin for the following muscles:

• long head of biceps femoris
• semitendinosus
• semimembranosus
• adductor magnus (shared origin)

Case 13.12

A Left hepatic artery

B Common hepatic artery

C Gastroepiploic artery

D Gastroduodenal artery

E Right hepatic artery

The gastroduodenal artery supplies the duodenum and then continues as the gastroepiploic artery which supplies the greater curve of the stomach.

Remember **LHS** for the major coeliac axis branches:

Left gastric, Hepatic and Splenic.

Case 13.13

A Right frontozygomatic suture

B Right greater wing of sphenoid

C Right superior orbital fissure

D Left foramen rotundum

E Left lesser wing of sphenoid

You should be able to recognise the fissures and foramina of the skull base, including the:

- **Greater and lesser wings of the sphenoid bone** – visible as two thin dense lines which cross each other in the superolateral aspect of the orbit
- **Superior orbital fissure** – evident as a tubular lucency in the medial aspect of the orbit
- **Foramen rotundum** – a well-defined rounded lucency with dense borders, projected over the maxillary antrum just below the inferior orbital rim. The maxillary division (V3) of the trigeminal (CN V) nerve passes through it.

Case 13.14

A Articular cartilage of the patella

B Posterior cruciate ligament

C Anterior cruciate ligament

D Patellar tendon

E Tibial tuberosity

The anterior cruciate ligament (ACL) inserts anteriorly on the tibia, whereas the posterior cruciate ligament (PCL) inserts posteriorly. Each has a different appearance on MRI, with the ACL being striated and the PCL returning homogeneously low signal.

The mnemonic 'drink ALe in the PM' will help you remember the relationship of the cruciate ligaments in the knee joint.

- Anterior cruciate is **L**ateral
- Posterior cruciate is **M**edial

The patellar tendon arises from the inferior pole of the patella and inserts into the tibial tuberosity.

Case 13.15

A Epiphysis of right humeral head

B Carina

C Left main bronchus

D Left atrium

E Right atrium

The carina is the point at which the trachea bifurcates into the left and right main bronchi. The left atrium lies below the carina, and as such, splaying of the carina is seen in the event of left atrial enlargement (e.g. in mitral valve disease). The right atrium forms the lower part of the right heart border and is typically obscured in cases of right middle lobe collapse or consolidation. The left ventricle forms the lower part of the left heart border. The right ventricle sits anteriorly and does not contribute to the heart borders as seen on a frontal radiograph.

Case 13.16

    A Anterior communicating artery (ACom)

    B Left anterior cerebral artery (ACA)

    C Right posterior cerebral artery (PCA)

    D Basilar artery (BA)

    E Petrous portion of the left internal carotid artery (ICA)

The circle of Willis is an anastomotic circle between the anterior and posterior cerebral circulations. It is formed by branches of the ICA and BA and forms a satellite configuration in the suprasellar cistern.

The circle comprises the following paired arteries:

- ACA – ICA branches
- ACom – ACA branch
- ICAs
- PCA – BA branches
- Posterior communicating arteries – middle cerebral artery branches

Case 13.17

    A Urinary bladder

    B Ossification centre of left femoral capital epiphysis

    C Urethra

    D Right obturator foramen

    E Right ilium

In a paediatric context, micturating cystourethrography is typically performed when investigating recurrent urinary tract infections. The urinary bladder is catheterised and contrast instilled in a retrograde fashion, with spot films taken (such as the image shown here) to assess for structural abnormalities (including ureterocoele). Once the bladder is full, the catheter is removed and imaging is performed during micturition to assess for vesicoureteric reflux, which is a potential cause of recurrent urinary tract infections. Vesicoureteric reflux will be seen as contrast which passes superiorly into the ureters and which may reach the pelvicalyceal systems, depending on severity.

Case 13.18

    A Right gluteus minimus muscle

    B Right piriformis muscle

    C Left inferior gluteal artery

    D Left internal iliac artery

    E Left external iliac artery

This is an axial view of a male pelvis taken during a CT angiogram examination. The external and internal iliac vessels are seen in the axial plane. Also note the inferior gluteal artery as it passes through the greater sciatic foramen to supply the muscles of the buttock. The piriformis muscle originates from the sacrum, exits via the greater sciatic foramen and attaches to the greater trochanter of the femur, acting as a lateral rotator of the hip.

Case 13.19

A Humerus

B Lamina

C Left coracoid process

D Blade of scapula

E Left clavicle

The purpose of the swimmer's view is to improve visualisation of the C7/T1 junction by ensuring that the humeral heads are projected away from the cervical spine, which is particularly important since a significant proportion of trauma to the cervicothoracic spine occurs at this level. Views like this may cause confusion but can still crop up in examinations. It is important to recognise the other structures that can appear on this view (including clavicle, humerus and scapula).

Case 13.20

A Segment II

B Segment I

C Segment VII

D Segment VIII

E Segment IVa

The Couinaud classification divides the liver anatomy into eight segments, all of which function independently (**Figure 13.1**). Each segment is centred on branches

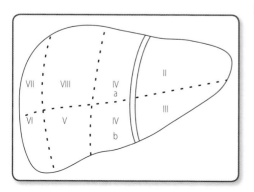

Figure 13.1 Segments of the liver.

of the portal vein, hepatic artery and bile duct. In the periphery of each segment, vascular outflow is provided via the hepatic veins.

- The right hepatic vein divides the right lobe into anterior and posterior segments
- The middle hepatic vein divides the liver into right and left lobes
- The left hepatic vein divides the left lobe into medial and lateral segments
- The portal vein divides the liver into upper and lower segments
- Segment IV is also divided to segments IVa and IVb
- Segment I is a posterior structure which drains directly into the IVC and is not seen on an anterior view
- Segments II, IVa, VII and VIII lie above the portal vein
- Segments III, IVb, V and VI lie below the portal vein

Chapter 14

Mock paper 14

20 cases to be answered in 75 minutes

Case 14.1

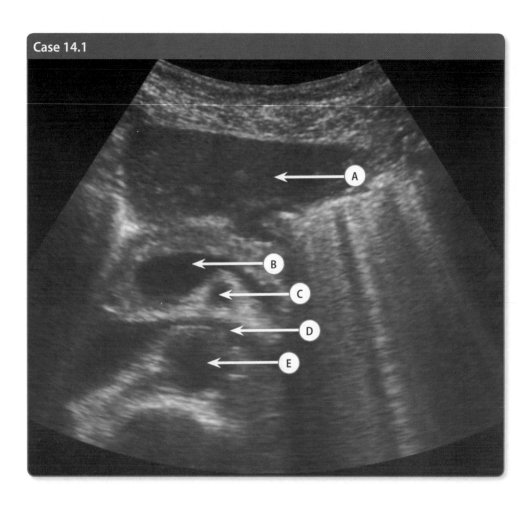

Case 14.1

QUESTION		WRITE YOUR ANSWER HERE
A	Name the structure labelled A.	
B	Name the structure labelled B.	
C	Name the structure labelled C.	
D	Name the structure labelled D.	
E	Name the structure labelled E.	

Case 14.2

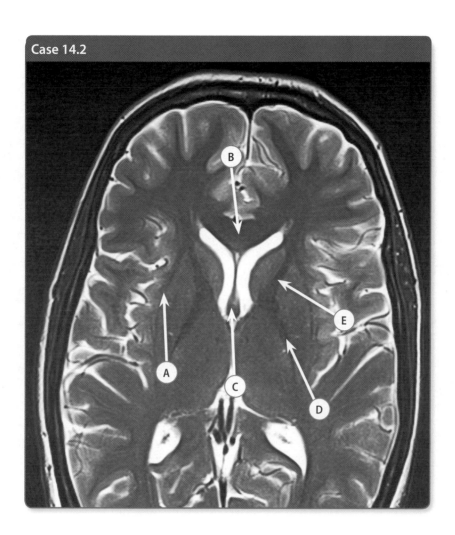

Case 14.2

QUESTION		WRITE YOUR ANSWER HERE
A	Name the structure labelled A.	
B	Name the structure labelled B.	
C	Name the structure labelled C.	
D	Name the structure labelled D.	
E	Name the structure labelled E.	

Case 14.3

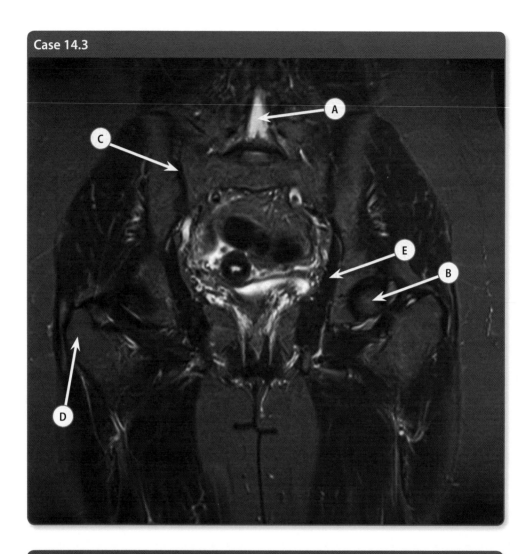

Case 14.3

QUESTION		WRITE YOUR ANSWER HERE
A	What accounts for the high signal labelled A?	
B	Name the structure labelled B.	
C	Name the structure labelled C.	
D	Name one muscle that inserts into the structure labelled D.	
E	Name the structure labelled E.	

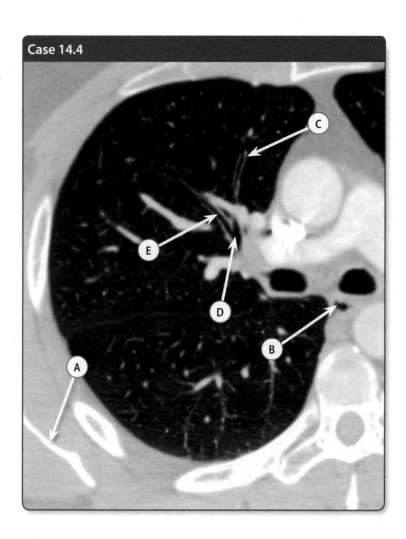

Case 14.4

QUESTION		WRITE YOUR ANSWER HERE
A	Name the structure labelled A.	
B	Name the structure labelled B.	
C	Name the structure labelled C	
D	Name the structure labelled D.	
E	Name the structure labelled E.	

Case 14.5

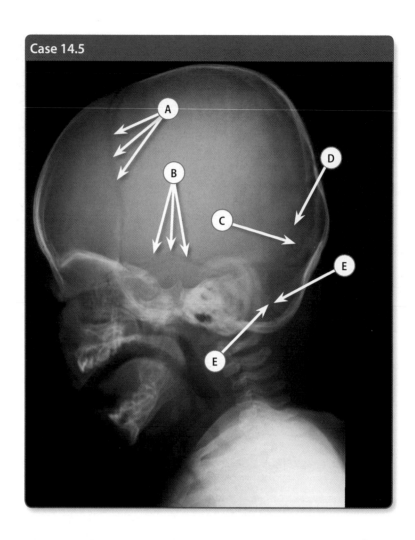

Case 14.5

QUESTION		WRITE YOUR ANSWER HERE
A	Name the structure labelled A.	
B	Name the structure labelled B.	
C	What osseous anatomical variant is labelled C?	
D	Name the structure labelled D.	
E	Name the structure labelled E.	

Case 14.6

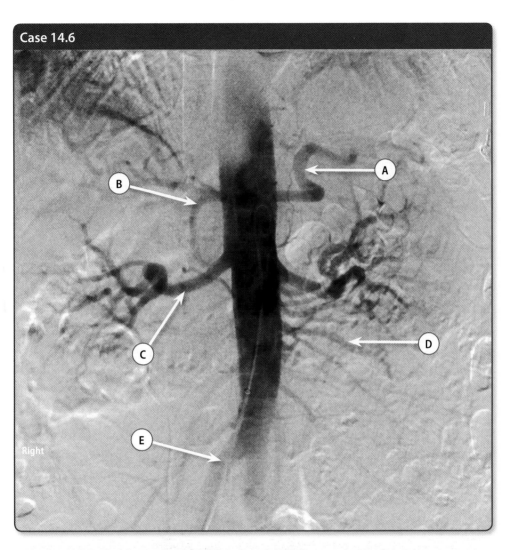

Case 14.6

QUESTION		WRITE YOUR ANSWER HERE
A	Name the structure labelled A.	
B	Name the structure labelled B.	
C	Name the structure labelled C.	
D	Name the structure labelled D.	
E	Name the structure labelled E.	

Case 14.7

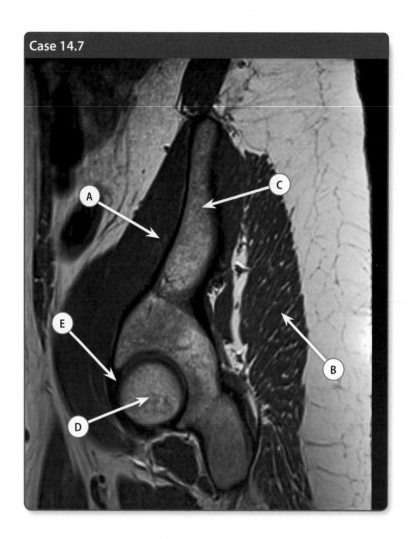

Case 14.7

QUESTION		WRITE YOUR ANSWER HERE
A	Name the structure labelled A.	
B	Name the structure labelled B.	
C	Name the structure labelled C.	
D	Name the structure labelled D.	
E	Name the structure labelled E.	

Case 14.8

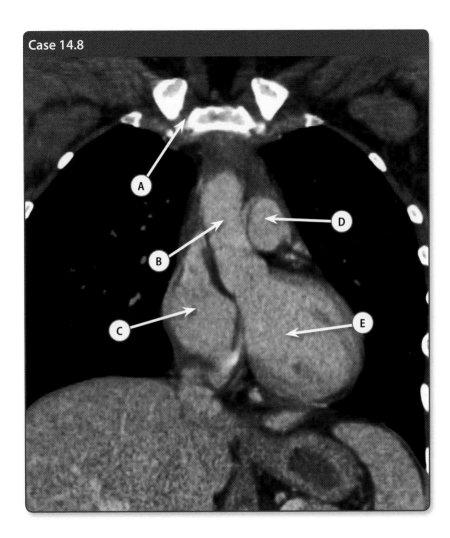

Case 14.8

QUESTION		WRITE YOUR ANSWER HERE
A	Name the structure labelled A.	
B	Name the structure labelled B.	
C	Name the chamber labelled C.	
D	Name the structure labelled D.	
E	Name the chamber labelled E.	

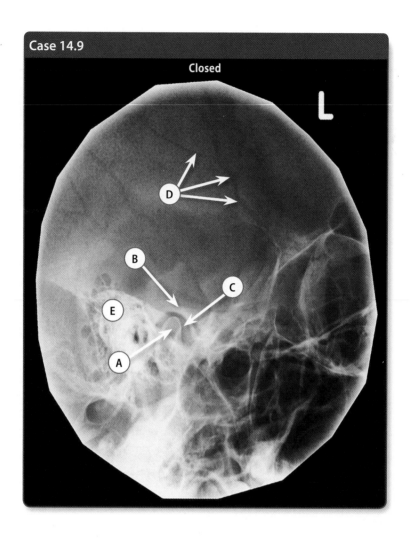

Case 14.9

Closed

L

Case 14.9

QUESTION		WRITE YOUR ANSWER HERE
A	Name the structure labelled A.	
B	Name the structure labelled B.	
C	Name the structure labelled C.	
D	Name the structure labelled D.	
E	Name the structure labelled E.	

Case 14.10

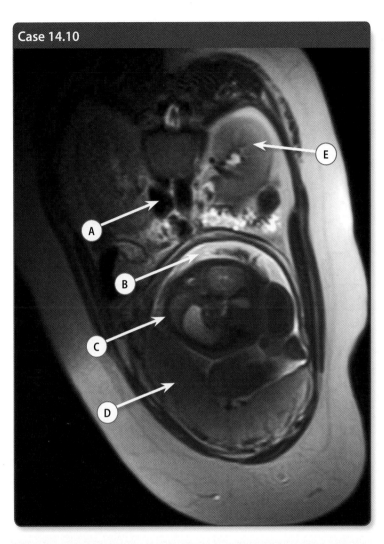

Case 14.10

QUESTION		WRITE YOUR ANSWER HERE
A	Name the structure labelled A.	
B	Name the structure labelled B.	
C	Name the structure labelled C.	
D	Name the structure labelled D.	
E	Name the structure labelled E.	

Case 14.11

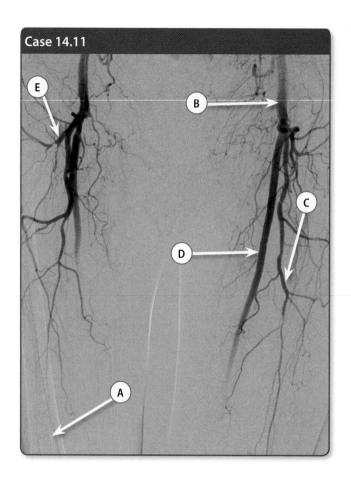

Case 14.11

QUESTION		WRITE YOUR ANSWER HERE
A	Name the structure labelled A.	
B	Name the structure labelled B.	
C	Name the structure labelled C.	
D	Name the structure labelled D.	
E	Name the structure labelled E.	

Case 14.12

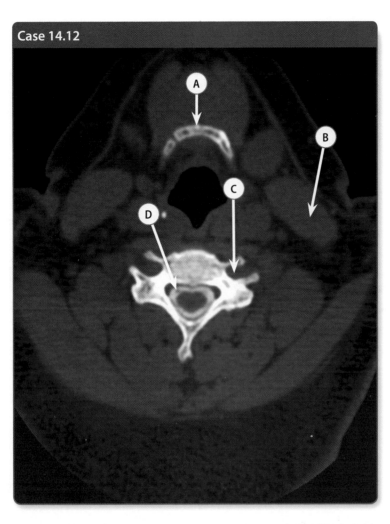

Case 14.12 Axial image at the level of C4

QUESTION		WRITE YOUR ANSWER HERE
A	Name the structure labelled A.	
B	Name the structure labelled B.	
C	Name the structure labelled C.	
D	Name the structure labelled D.	
E	From what investigation is this image taken?	

Case 14.13

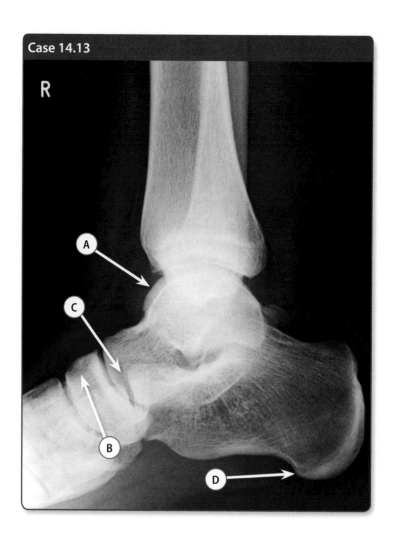

R

Case 14.13

QUESTION		WRITE YOUR ANSWER HERE
A	Name the structure labelled A.	
B	Name the structure labelled B.	
C	Name the structure labelled C.	
D	What structure attaches to D?	
E	What accessory ossicle is present?	

Case 14.14

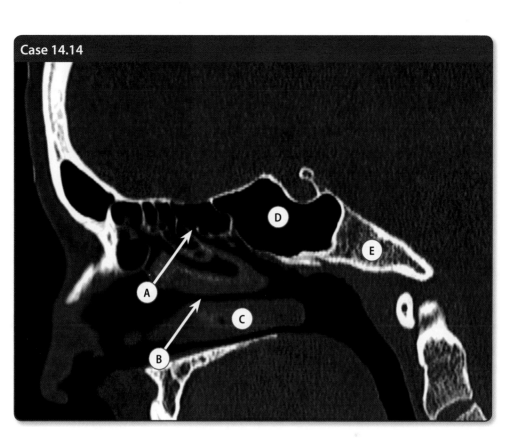

Case 14.14

QUESTION		WRITE YOUR ANSWER HERE
A	Name the space labelled A.	
B	Name the space labelled B.	
C	Name the structure labelled C.	
D	Name the structure labelled D.	
E	Name the structure labelled E.	

Case 14.15

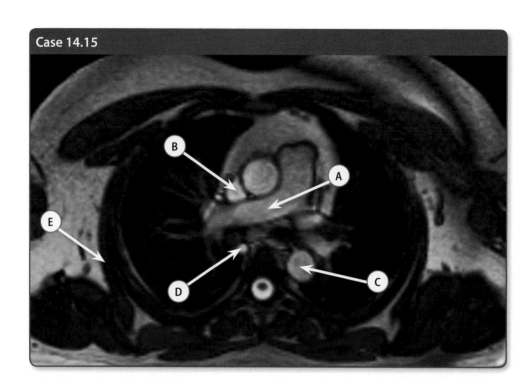

Case 14.15

QUESTION		WRITE YOUR ANSWER HERE
A	Name the structure labelled A.	
B	Name the structure labelled B.	
C	Name the structure labelled C.	
D	Name the structure labelled D.	
E	Name the structure labelled E.	

Case 14.16

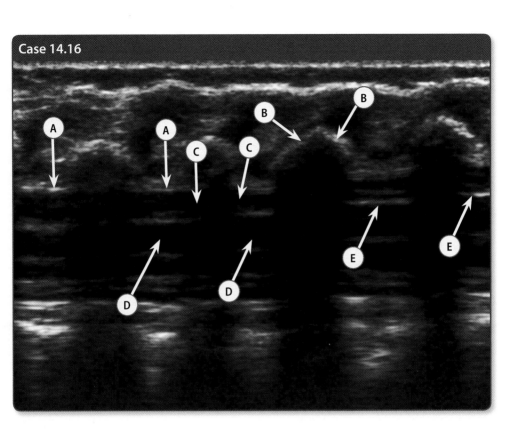

Case 14.16 Ultrasound of the thoracic cord of a neonate

QUESTION		WRITE YOUR ANSWER HERE
A	Name the meningeal layer(s) labelled A.	
B	Name the structure labelled B.	
C	Name the structure labelled C.	
D	Name the structure labelled D.	
E	Name the meningeal layer(s) labelled E.	

Case 14.17

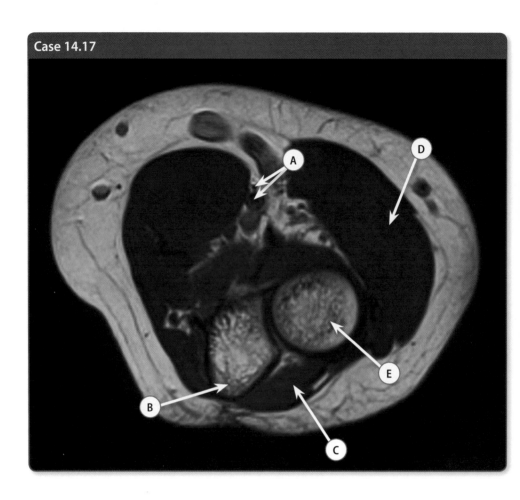

Case 14.17

QUESTION		WRITE YOUR ANSWER HERE
A	Name the structure labelled A.	
B	Name the structure labelled B.	
C	Name the structure labelled C.	
D	Name the structure labelled D.	
E	Name the structure labelled E.	

Case 14.18

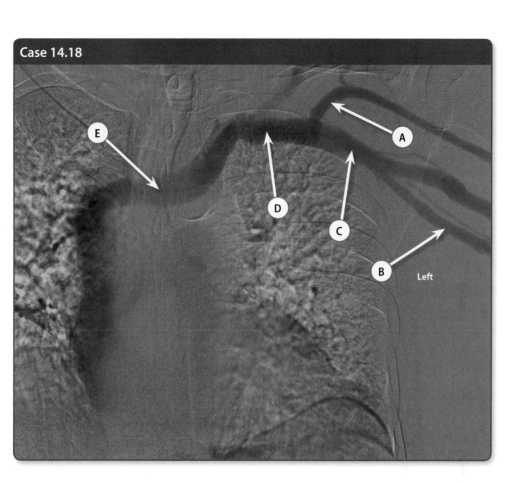

Case 14.18

QUESTION		WRITE YOUR ANSWER HERE
A	Name the structure labelled A.	
B	Name the structure labelled B.	
C	Name the structure labelled C.	
D	Name the structure labelled D.	
E	Name the structure labelled E.	

Case 14.19

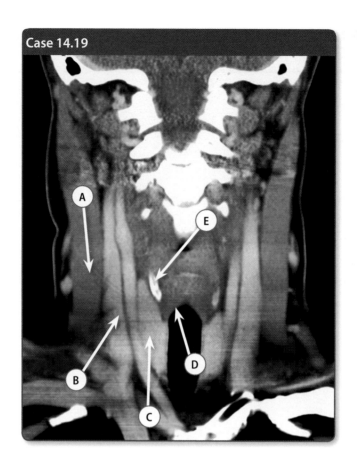

Case 14.19

QUESTION		WRITE YOUR ANSWER HERE
A	Name the structure labelled A.	
B	Name the structure labelled B.	
C	Name the structure labelled C.	
D	Name the structure labelled D.	
E	Name the structure labelled E.	

Case 14.20

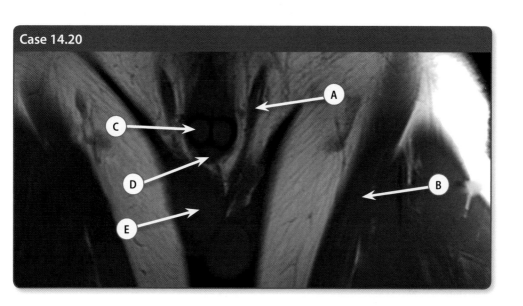

Case 14.20

QUESTION		WRITE YOUR ANSWER HERE
A	Name the structure labelled A.	
B	Name the structure labelled B.	
C	Name the structure labelled C.	
D	Name the structure labelled D.	
E	Name the structure labelled E.	

Answers

Case 14.1

A Left lobe of the liver

B Portal venous confluence

C Superior mesenteric artery

D Left renal vein

E Aorta

The left lobe of the liver is visualised at the top of the picture (A). The bright streakiness to the right of the image is caused by gas in the gastric lumen.

The portal venous confluence is formed by the splenic and superior mesenteric veins.

The course of the left renal vein is clearly demonstrated, running anterior to the abdominal aorta and posterior to the superior mesenteric artery.

Case 14.2

A Right external capsule

B Genu of corpus callosum

C Fornix

D Posterior limb of left internal capsule

E Anterior limb of left internal capsule

There are two main types of cerebral white matter tracts:

- **Transverse** (commissural) – linking paired structures across the midline. The corpus callosum is the largest commissural tract and is divided into four parts (from anterior to posterior): rostrum, genu, corpus and splenium. A good way of remembering this is that the genu (Latin for knee) points anteriorly.
- **Descending** – contain two pathways: the corticospinal, connecting the cerebral grey matter with the spinal cord; and the corticobulbar, between the cortex and motor nuclei in the brainstem. There are three main stations (from cranial to caudal): centrum semiovale, corona radiata and internal capsule.

Case 14.3

A Cerebrospinal fluid within the thecal sac

B Head of left femur

C Right sacroiliac joint

D Right gluteus medius or minimus muscle

E Left obturator internus muscle

The greater trochanter of the femur serves as the insertion site for both the gluteus minimus and gluteus medius muscles. The lesser trochanter is the insertion site for the iliopsoas tendon.

The paired obturator internus and obturator externus muscles may be easily remembered from their descriptors, with internus being inside the pelvis and externus being outwith the pelvis.

Case 14.4

A Blade of right scapula

B Oesophagus

C Medial segment bronchus of middle lobe

D Middle lobe bronchus

E Lateral segment bronchus of middle lobe

The right main bronchus (RMB) is wider, shorter and more vertical than the left main bronchus, which accounts for the greater tendency for aspirated material to pass down the RMB. The right upper lobe bronchus is the first lobar bronchus to branch off the RMB, which continues as the bronchus intermedius. The bronchus intermedius terminates as the middle and lower lobe bronchi.

This question requires that you understand the bronchopulmonary segments of the middle lobe. The middle lobe comprises lateral and medial bronchopulmonary segments.

Case 14.5

A Coronal suture

B Temporosquamal suture

C Wormian bone

D Lambdoid suture

E Occipitomastoid suture

Knowledge of the normal anatomy of the infant skull is vital to minimise the risk of confusing a normal suture for a fracture. Anatomy of the sutures is also of relevance in the assessment of craniosynostosis, when there is either symmetrical or asymmetrical premature sutural fusion which gives rise to an abnormally shaped calvarium. Wormian bones are usually a normal variant, most frequently located in the lambdoid suture. However, if numerous (greater than 10) or excessively large, they can be a marker of pathological processes such as osteogenesis imperfecta or pyknodysostosis.

Case 14.6

A Splenic artery

B Gastroduodenal artery

C Right renal artery

D Jejunal branch of superior mesenteric artery

E Right common iliac artery

The coeliac axis arises from the abdominal aorta at the level of T12 and almost immediately trifurcates into the splenic, left gastric and common hepatic arteries.

The right gastric and gastroduodenal arteries are branches of the common hepatic artery. The common hepatic artery then becomes the hepatic artery proper and further divides to give branches to the gallbladder (cystic artery) and lobar branches to the liver.

Variant anatomy is very common here and the hepatic artery and its branches may arise from the aorta or superior mesenteric artery.

Case 14.7

A Iliacus muscle

B Gluteus maximus muscle

C Ilium

D Femoral head

E Anterior superior acetabular labrum

MR imaging of the hip allows adequate visualisation of the labrum. Optimal evaluation is with MR arthrography, which involves direct injection of contrast into the joint under fluoroscopy guidance followed by acquisition of MRIs. It is important to remember that the acetabulum is a three-dimensional structure, hence different planar acquisitions allow evaluation of different aspects of the labrum:

- Axial – posterior and anterior labrum
- Sagittal – superior and inferior labrum
- Coronal – lateral labrum

The labrum, a cartilaginous structure, returns low signal intensity on all MR sequences – remember, fatty marrow is high signal on T1- weighted images.

Iliacus originates from the iliac blade and runs on the anterior surface of the ilium, where it conjoins with psoas major to form the iliopsoas tendon.

Case 14.8

A Right sternoclavicular joint

B Ascending aorta

C Right atrium

D Pulmonary trunk

E Left ventricle

The papillary muscles are evident in the cavity of the left ventricle. There are two papillary muscles in the left ventricle and three in the right ventricle. They attach to the cusps of the mitral and tricuspid valves respectively and prevent regurgitation of ventricular blood into the atria during systole.

The aortic valve is normally tricuspid but is congenitally bicuspid in 1% of individuals. This abnormal valve is more prone to aortic stenosis.

Case 14.9

A Left mandibular condyle

B Glenoid fossa of the left temporal bone

C Left temporomandibular joint (TMJ)

D Grooves for middle meningeal artery branches

E Mastoid portion of the left temporal bone

The TMJ is a synovial joint formed by the mandible and the temporal bone, lying anterior to the external acoustic meatus. It consists of the following parts:

- mandibular condyle
- glenoid fossa of the temporal bone
- joint capsule
- articular disc
- ligaments
- lateral pterygoid plate.

MRI is the modality of choice for assessing the TMJ. However, structures including the mandibular condyle and the glenoid fossa of the temporal bone are readily visible on plain radiographs.

Case 14.10

A Maternal inferior vena cava

B Amniotic fluid

C Fetus

D Placenta

E Maternal left kidney

This is a fetal MRI in the axial plane during the third trimester. Fetal MRI can be used to further visualise abnormalities detected on US. The fetal sac, fetus, placenta and amniotic fluid are nicely visualised.

Fetal MRI has appeared in the anatomy section of the first FRCR examination. It is important to familiarise yourselves with a few examples and be able to identify important structures such as the fetal poles, amnion, placenta and umbilical cord. You might also be asked to estimate the trimester of gestation. Bear this in mind when revising and don't be too worried or afraid of it. You will almost certainly be expected to identify some maternal structures as well.

Case 14.11

A Right femur

B Left common femoral artery

C Left profunda femoris artery

D Left superficial femoral artery

E Right lateral circumflex femoral artery

The external iliac artery becomes the common femoral artery (CFA) at the level of the inguinal ligament. The CFA bifurcates into:

- profunda femoris artery
- superficial femoral artery

The profunda femoris artery has lateral and medial circumflex femoral artery branches along with multiple horizontal perforators.

Case 14.12

A Body of hyoid

B Left sternocleidomastoid muscle

C Left foramen transversarium

D Right C4 ventral nerve root

E CT myelogram

CT myelography may be performed when MRI is contraindicated, to evaluate nerve roots and assess for the presence of intervertebral disc disease. Contrast is administered into the thecal sac and outlines the nerve roots. The ventral spinal roots carry only somatic motor fibres in the cervical spine, but will also carry sympathetic fibres from the T1–L2 levels and parasympathetic fibres from the S2–S4 levels. Afferent sensory fibres (somatic and visceral) are carried along the dorsal nerve roots. The dorsal and ventral nerve roots form the mixed spinal nerve within the intervertebral canal.

Case 14.13

A Dome of right talus

B Right navicular bone

C Head of right talus

D Right plantar fascia

E Os trigonum

Accessory ossicles of the foot are seen in approximately one in five people. There are at least 15 known accessory ossicles, the most commonly seen being:

- os tibiale externum (accessory navicular)
- os fibulare (peroneum)
- os trigonum
- os supranaviculare

Case 14.14

A Posterior ethmoid ostium

B Middle meatus

C Inferior turbinate (concha)

D Sphenoid sinus

E Clivus

Each lateral wall of the nasal cavity consist of three turbinates (conchae). These are osteocartilaginous projections which are covered by mucosa and separated by spaces known as meati:

- **Superior meatus** – site of drainage of the posterior ethmoidal cells
- **Middle meatus** – site of drainage of the anterior osteomeatal complex, a common route of drainage from the anterior and middle ethmoid air cells, maxillary and frontal sinuses
- **Inferior meatus** – site of drainage of the nasolacrimal duct

Case 14.15

A Right pulmonary artery

B Superior vena cava

C Descending thoracic aorta

D Azygos vein

E Right serratus anterior muscle

The right pulmonary artery lies horizontal at this level, passing posterior to the ascending aorta and the superior vena cava and anterior to the two major bronchi and the oesophagus. There is a fair amount of anterior pericardial fat (shown as a white crescent anterior to the great vessels), the same appearance as the fat in the axillae and breasts. Note that a trace amount of pericardial fluid (up to 5 mL) is often visible on both MRI and ultrasound of the heart and is a normal finding.

Case 14.16

A Dura mater

B Spinous process

C Subarachnoid space

D Spinal cord

E Pia and arachnoid mater

It is possible to visualise the spinal cord using ultrasound in the first few months of life, whilst posterior spinal arches are incompletely ossified. The spinal cord itself is seen on longitudinal ultrasound as a hypoechoic tubular structure with a central echogenic stripe corresponding to the central canal. The echogenic line on either side of the cord represents the pia and arachnoid mater, which lie very close to each other and cannot be distinguished separately on ultrasound. The hypoechoic cerebrospinal fluid-filled subarachnoid space lies between the arachnoid mater and the dura mater (also seen as an echogenic stripe). Dense acoustic shadowing is seen from the spinous processes.

Case 14.17

A Brachial vessels

B Olecranon of ulna

C Anconeus muscle

D Brachioradialis muscle

E Head of radius

The round osseous structure on this image should be easily identified as the head of radius (E). Having identified the radial head, the remaining labels can be established methodically:

- (B) the olecranon forms the posterior part of the trochlear notch of the proximal ulna
- (C) anconeus lies posterior to the radius
- (D) brachioradialis is the most anterior lateral muscle of the proximal forearm

The brachial vessels most commonly consist of a single artery with paired brachial veins.

Case 14.18

A Left cephalic vein

B Left basilic vein

C Left axillary vein

D Left subclavian vein

E Left brachiocephalic vein

Venous drainage of the arm is highly variable. The most constant veins are the cephalic, basilic and brachial veins. The brachial and basilic veins unite to form the axillary vein. The subclavian vein is formed by the confluence of the axillary and cephalic veins. The internal jugular vein joins the subclavian vein to form the brachiocephalic vein.

Case 14.19

A Right sternocleidomastoid muscle

B Right internal jugular vein

C Right lobe of the thyroid gland

D Right true vocal cord

E Thyroid cartilage

The two lobes of the thyroid gland lie on either side of the trachea and appear chevron-shaped on coronal imaging. The thyroid gland appears relatively dense on non-enhanced CT due to the presence of iodine. The thyroid is directly related to the larynx medially and the carotid space (containing the vagus nerve (CN X), common carotid artery and internal jugular vein) laterally.

Case 14.20

A Left spermatic cord

B Left sartorius muscle

C Right corpus cavernosum

D Corpus spongiosum

E Right testis

The spermatic cord (A) descends to the testis after it exits the superficial inguinal ring. The spermatic cord is covered by the external spermatic fascia, cremasteric muscle/fascia and internal spermatic fascia. It conveys the vas deferens, nerves, arteries, lymphatics and pampiniform venous plexus.

Chapter 15

Mock paper 15

20 cases to be answered in 75 minutes

Case 15.1

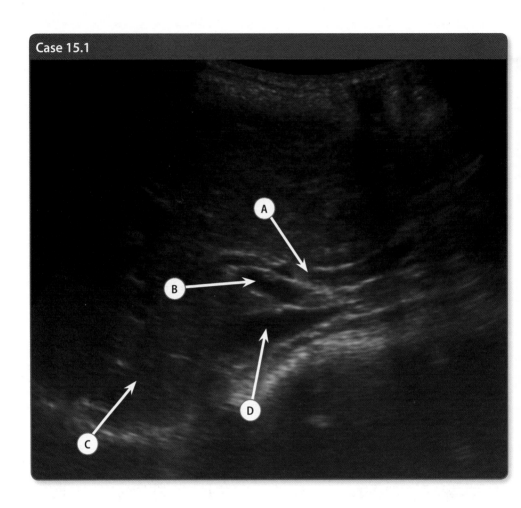

Case 15.1

QUESTION		WRITE YOUR ANSWER HERE
A	Name the structure labelled A.	
B	Name the structure labelled B.	
C	Name the structure labelled C.	
D	Name the structure labelled D.	
E	What is the upper limit of normal for the common bile duct diameter?	

Case 15.2

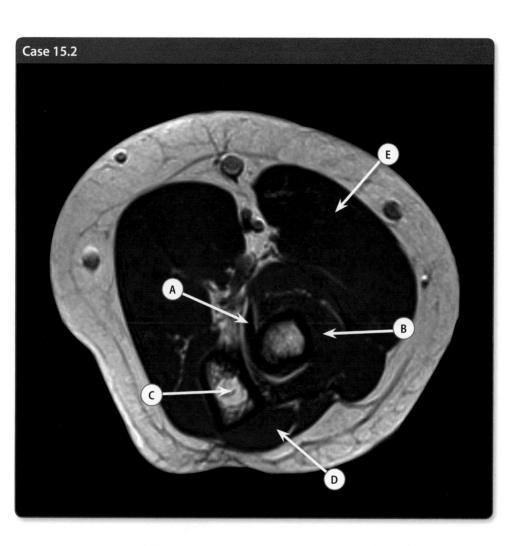

Case 15.2

QUESTION		WRITE YOUR ANSWER HERE
A	Name the structure labelled A.	
B	Name the structure labelled B.	
C	Name the structure labelled C.	
D	Name the structure labelled D.	
E	Name the structure labelled E.	

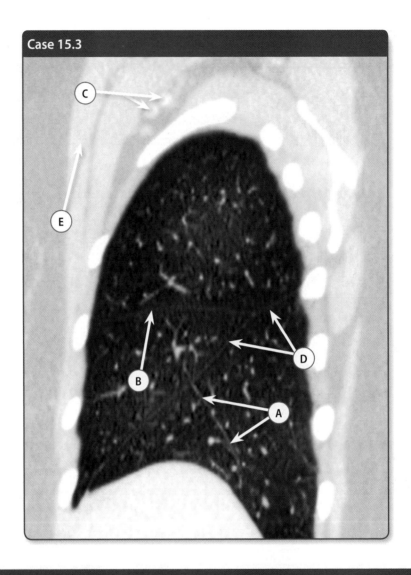

Case 15.3

QUESTION		WRITE YOUR ANSWER HERE
A	Name the structure labelled A.	
B	Name the structure labelled B.	
C	Name the structure labelled C.	
D	Name the structure labelled D.	
E	Name the structure labelled E.	

Case 15.4

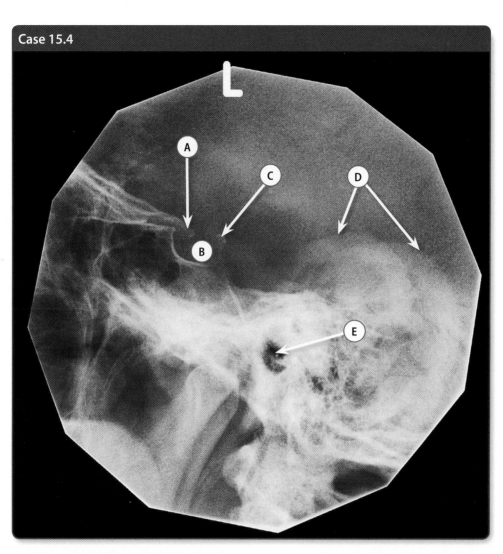

Case 15.4

QUESTION		WRITE YOUR ANSWER HERE
A	Name the structure labelled A.	
B	Name the structure labelled B.	
C	Name the structure labelled C	
D	Name the structure labelled D.	
E	Name the structure labelled E.	

Case 15.5

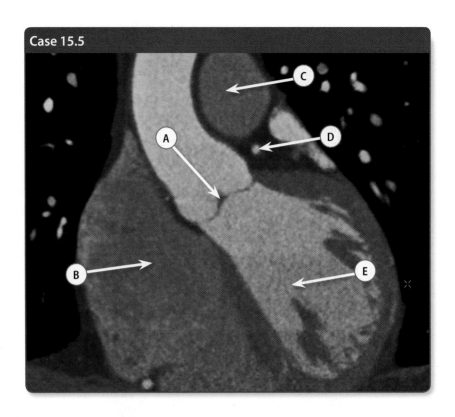

Case 15.5

QUESTION		WRITE YOUR ANSWER HERE
A	Name the structure labelled A.	
B	Name the chamber labelled B.	
C	Name the structure labelled C.	
D	Name the structure labelled D.	
E	Name the chamber labelled E.	

Case 15.6

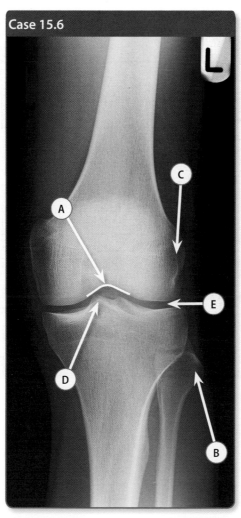

Case 15.6

QUESTION		WRITE YOUR ANSWER HERE
A	Name the outlined structure labelled A.	
B	Name the structure labelled B.	
C	Name the structure labelled C.	
D	Name the structure labelled D.	
E	Name the structure that predominantly occupies the space labelled E.	

Case 15.7

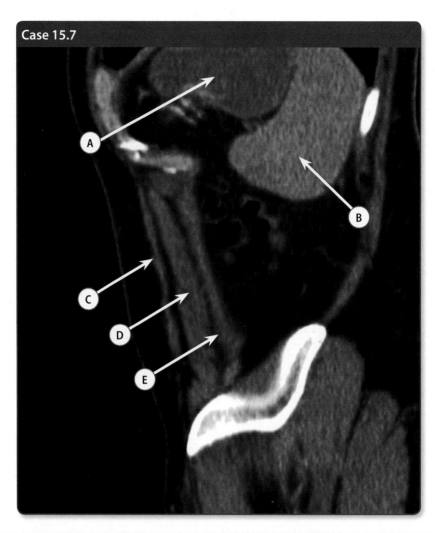

Case 15.7

QUESTION		WRITE YOUR ANSWER HERE
A	Name the structure labelled A.	
B	Name the structure labelled B.	
C	Name the structure labelled C.	
D	Name the structure labelled D.	
E	Name the structure labelled E.	

Case 15.8

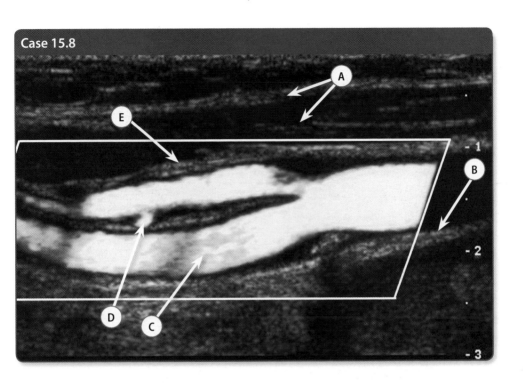

Case 15.8

QUESTION		WRITE YOUR ANSWER HERE
A	Name the structure labelled A.	
B	Name the structure labelled B.	
C	Name the structure labelled C.	
D	Name the structure labelled D.	
E	Name the structure labelled E.	

Case 15.9

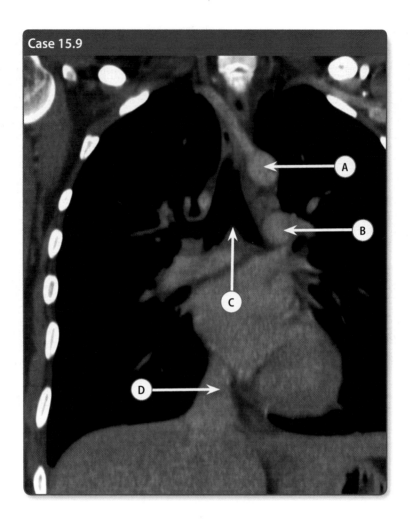

Case 15.9

	QUESTION	WRITE YOUR ANSWER HERE
A	Name the structure labelled A.	
B	Name the structure labelled B.	
C	Name the structure labelled C.	
D	Name the structure labelled D.	
E	Which anatomical variant is present on this image?	

Case 15.10

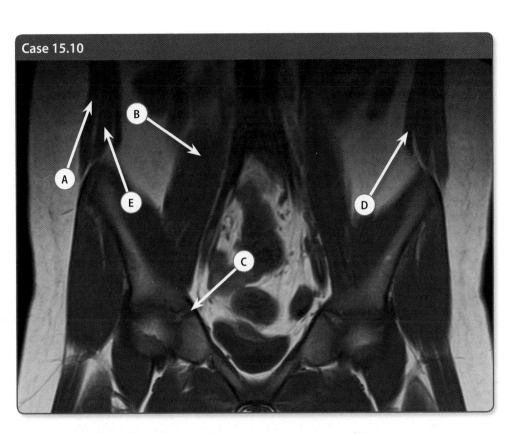

Case 15.10

QUESTION	WRITE YOUR ANSWER HERE
A Name the structure labelled A.	
B Name the structure labelled B.	
C Name the structure labelled C.	
D Name the structure labelled D.	
E Name the structure labelled E.	

Case 15.11

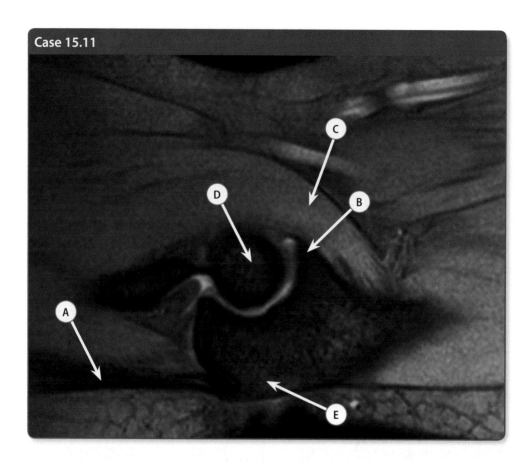

Case 15.11

QUESTION		WRITE YOUR ANSWER HERE
A	Name the structure labelled A.	
B	Name the structure labelled B.	
C	Name the structure labelled C.	
D	Name the structure labelled D.	
E	Name the structure labelled E.	

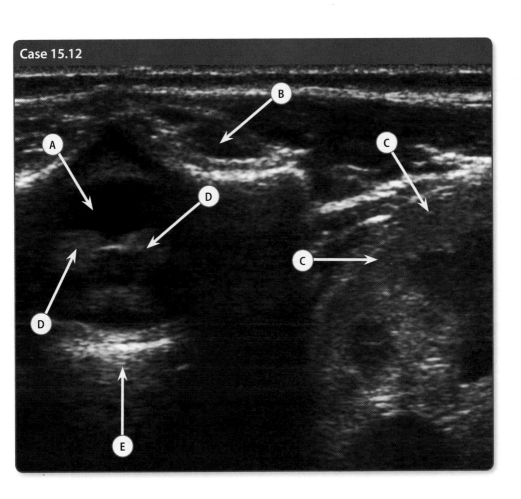

Case 15.12

Case 15.12 Axial ultrasound of a neonatal conus medullaris

QUESTION		WRITE YOUR ANSWER HERE
A	Name the space labelled A.	
B	Name the structure labelled B.	
C	Name the structure labelled C.	
D	Name the structure labelled D.	
E	Name the structure labelled E.	

Case 15.13

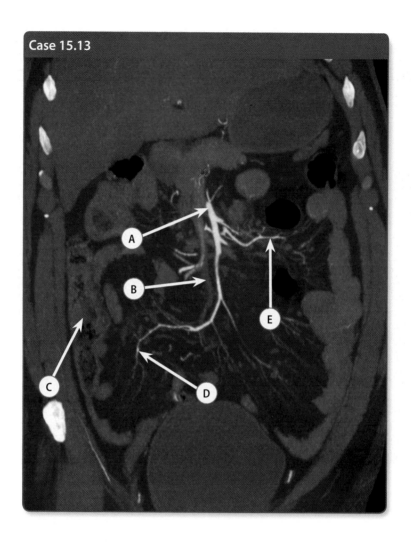

Case 15.13

QUESTION		WRITE YOUR ANSWER HERE
A	Name the structure labelled A.	
B	Name the structure labelled B.	
C	Name the structure labelled C.	
D	Name the structure labelled D.	
E	Name the structure labelled E.	

Case 15.14

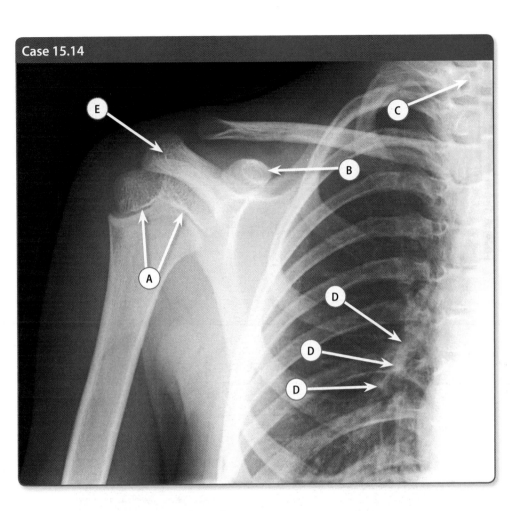

Case 15.14

QUESTION		WRITE YOUR ANSWER HERE
A	Name the structure labelled A.	
B	Name the structure labelled B.	
C	Name the structure labelled C.	
D	Name the structure labelled D.	
E	Name the structure labelled E.	

Case 15.15

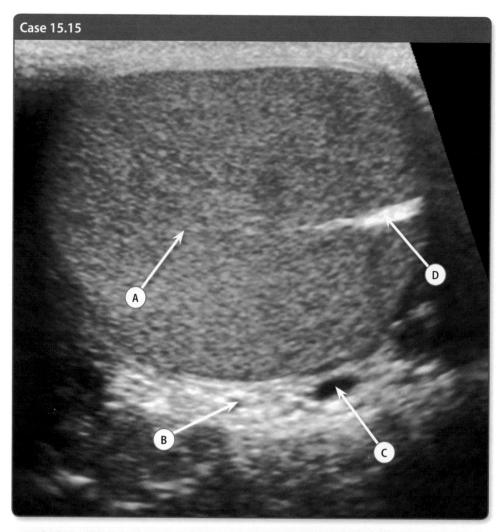

Case 15.15

QUESTION		WRITE YOUR ANSWER HERE
A	Name the structure labelled A.	
B	Name the structure labelled B.	
C	Name the structure labelled C.	
D	Name the structure labelled D.	
E	Where does the left testicular vein drain to?	

Case 15.16

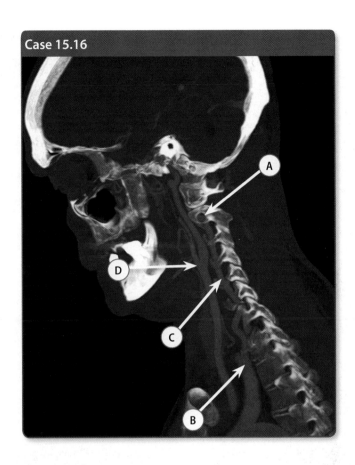

Case 15.16		
QUESTION		**WRITE YOUR ANSWER HERE**
A	Name the structure labelled A.	
B	Name the structure labelled B.	
C	Name the structure labelled C.	
D	Name the structure labelled D.	
E	What is the first branch of the external carotid artery called?	

Case 15.17

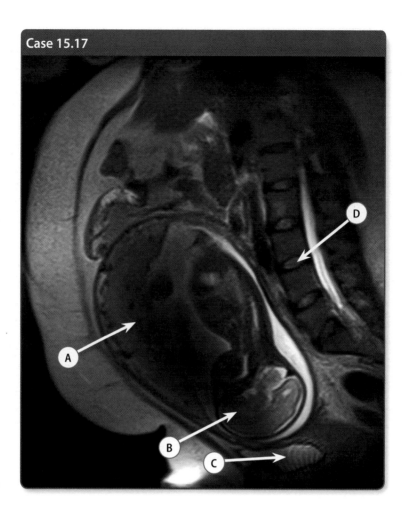

Case 15.17

QUESTION		WRITE YOUR ANSWER HERE
A	Name the structure labelled A.	
B	Name the structure labelled B.	
C	Name the structure labelled C.	
D	Name the structure labelled D.	
E	In which trimester of preganacy was this investigation performed?	

Case 15.18

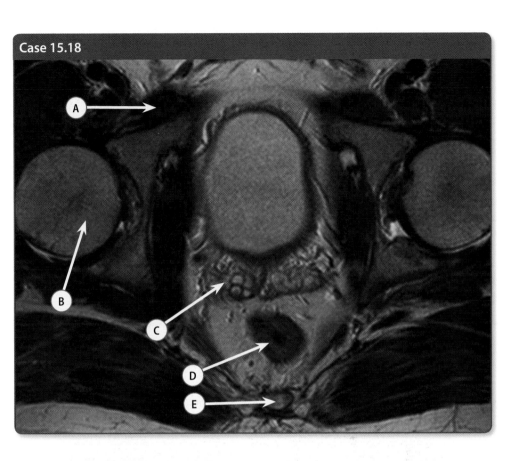

Case 15.18

QUESTION		WRITE YOUR ANSWER HERE
A	Name the structure labelled A.	
B	Name the structure labelled B.	
C	Name the structure labelled C.	
D	Name the structure labelled D.	
E	Name the structure labelled E.	

Case 15.19

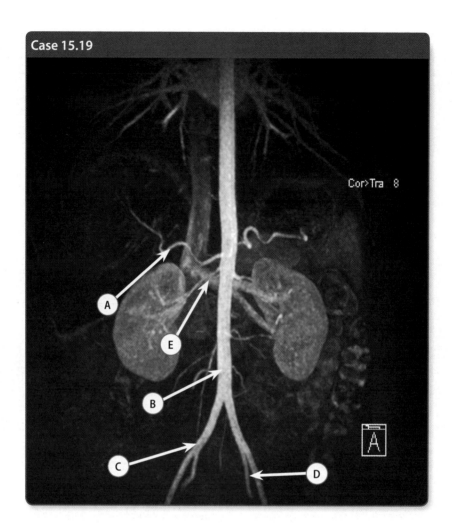

Case 15.19

QUESTION		WRITE YOUR ANSWER HERE
A	Name the structure labelled A.	
B	Name the structure labelled B.	
C	Name the structure labelled C.	
D	Name the structure labelled D.	
E	What anatomical variant is labelled E?	

Case 15.20

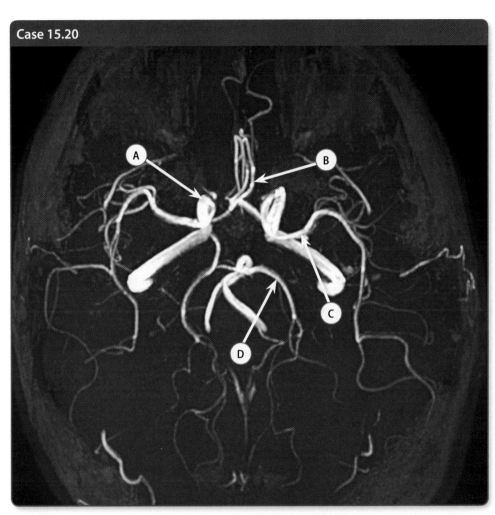

Case 15.20

QUESTION		WRITE YOUR ANSWER HERE
A	Name the structure labelled A.	
B	Name the structure labelled B.	
C	Name the structure labelled C.	
D	Name the structure labelled D.	
E	Which anatomical variant is present on this image?	

Answers

Case 15.1

A Common bile duct

B Portal vein

C Right liver lobe

D Inferior vena cava

E 6 mm

This example demonstrates the relationship of the portal vein to the inferior vena cava and common hepatic duct, with the portal vein located between those two structures. Note the position of the common bile duct anterior to the portal vein at the porta hepatis. The normal size of the common bile duct in a healthy biliary system is up to 6 mm, but may increase by up to 9 mm in elderly patients and post-cholecystectomy.

Case 15.2

A Tendon of biceps brachii muscle

B Supinator muscle

C Ulna

D Anconeus muscle

E Brachioradialis muscle

Axial anatomy of the forearm may be difficult. Here are a few aide-mémoires to help you with memorising some key structures.

- the supinator muscle wraps around the proximal radius
- anteriorly, the most lateral muscle of the proximal forearm is brachioradialis
- anteriorly, the most medial muscle of the proximal forearm is pronator teres
- the anconeus muscle is seen posterior to supinator and is wedged between the proximal ulna and radius posteriorly.

Case 15.3

A Right superior accessory fissure

B Horizontal fissure

C Right subclavian vessels

D Right oblique fissure

E Right pectoralis major muscle

The superior accessory fissure is seen in up to 4% of chest CT scans and separates the superior segment from the basal segments of the right lower lobe. Other accessory fissures include the inferior accessory fissure and the azygos lobe fissure.

A left minor fissure is present in approximately 8% of individuals, but can only be identified on chest radiographs in 1.6% of patients. The left minor fissure, when present, typically separates the lingula from the rest of the left upper lobe.

Case 15.4

A Anterior clinoid process

B Pituitary fossa

C Posterior clinoid process

D Pinnae of ears

E Left external auditory canal

The pituitary fossa (sella turcica, meaning Turkish saddle) is a saddle-shaped depression in the superior portion of the sphenoid bone in the middle cranial fossa. The saddle of the sella, in which the pituitary gland sits, is called the hypophyseal fossa. The tuberculum sellae is a small bony bulge situated anterior to the hypophyseal fossa. The dorsum sellae forms the posterior boundary of the saddle, terminating laterally as the posterior clinoid processes. The anterior clinoid processes are frontal continuations of the sella.

Case 15.5

A Aortic valve

B Right atrium

C Pulmonary trunk /main pulmonary artery

D Left coronary artery

E Left ventricle

The left coronary artery arises from the left posterior aortic sinus and courses posterior to the pulmonary trunk in the left atrioventricular groove, in which it bifurcates into the left circumflex artery and the left anterior descending artery.

Case 15.6

A Intercondylar notch of the left femur

B Head of left fibula

C Lateral condyle of left femur

D Medial prominence of tibial spine (intercondyloid eminence)

E Left lateral meniscus

Four bones are evident on the frontal knee radiograph:

1.   distal femur

2.   proximal tibia – medial

3.   proximal fibula – lateral

4.   patella – superimposed onto the distal femur. Depending on the beam angle, you may see the inferior patellar pole projected over the intercondylar notch of the distal femur

Remember the fibuLA lies LAteral to the tibia.

Case 15.7

A Stomach

B Spleen

C Left external oblique muscle

D Left internal oblique muscle

E Left transversus abdominis muscle

The stomach has been filled with water, hence its distended appearance, with the left hemidiaphragm lying just above it. Parasagittal views (both CT and MRI) are ideal imaging tools for assessing diaphragmatic disease including congenital and acquired hernias, eventrations and traumatic ruptures. The diaphragm also has variable anatomical appearances and this projection will help in assessing the presence of multiple slips.

Case 15.8

A Sternocleidomastoid muscle fibres

B Intima of the common carotid artery

C Internal carotid artery

D Ascending pharyngeal artery

E Adventitia of the external carotid artery

Ultrasound examination of the carotid arteries is a non-invasive procedure used as a first line assessment of the severity of the carotid narrowing. This B-mode image is used for assessment of the morphology of the arterial lumen. The normal carotid artery produces two parallel echoes in B-mode imaging, which correspond to the internal and external layers of the wall, the intima and adventitia respectively. The hypoechoic stripe between these layers represents the media.

External carotid artery (ECA) gives off several branches in the neck, the second one being the ascending pharyngeal artery. Remember that the internal carotid artery lies deeper to the external carotid artery and does not give off any branches in the neck.

Case 15.9

A Arch of aorta

B Pulmonary trunk

C Carina

D Inferior vena cava

E Aberrant right subclavian artery

An aberrant right subclavian artery is a common anatomical variant of the aortic arch. The aberrant artery usually arises distal to the left subclavian artery from a dilated segment of aorta called the 'diverticulum of Kommerell'. It usually courses posterior to the oesophagus and can lead to oesophageal compression, thus causing dysphagia (otherwise known as 'dysphagia lusoria').

Case 15.10

A Right external oblique muscle

B Right psoas major muscle

C Right triradiate cartilage

D Left transversus abdominis muscle

E Right internal oblique muscle

The musculature of the abdominal wall comprises the paired anterior rectus abdominis muscles and lateral wall musculature. The muscles of the lateral wall comprise, from deepest to most superficial, **TIE**:

- **T**ransversus abdominis
- **I**nternal oblique
- **E**xternal oblique

These muscles can be easily seen on both MRI and CT examinations.

Case 15.11

A Triceps brachii tendon

B Coronoid process of ulna

C Brachialis

D Trochlea of humerus

E Olecranon of ulna

This sagittal MRI of the medial aspect of the elbow shows the articulation between the distal humerus and proximal ulna. The trochlea of the distal humerus lies within the trochlear notch of the ulna, the anterior boundary of which is formed by the coronoid process and the posterior boundary by the olecranon.

In elbow extension, the olecranon fills the olecranon fossa of the distal humerus posteriorly. In flexion, the coronoid process fills the coronoid fossa of the humerus anteriorly.

The brachialis muscle is unique in that the bulk of its muscle is seen to cross the elbow joint.

Case 15.12

A Subarachnoid space

B Left erector spinae muscle

C Left kidney

D Spinal cord

E Vertebral body

The conus medullaris is the expansion at the caudal end of the spinal cord. In neonates, the tip of the conus medullaris typically lies between L1 and L2. A low-lying conus medullaris (i.e. below the level of L2–3) suggests spinal dysraphism, with associated tethering of an abnormally thickened filum terminale. The filum terminale is a condensation of pia mater that continues caudally from the tip of the conus medullaris to attach to the dorsal aspect of the first coccygeal segment. The central canal of the cord continues within the filum terminale for 5–6 cm. The filum terminale should normally measure no more than 2 mm in thickness.

Case 15.13

A Superior mesenteric artery (SMA)

B Superior mesenteric vein

C Ascending colon

D Ileocolic branch

E Jejunal branch

The SMA and major branches are depicted. Note the normal anatomical position of the superior mesenteric vein (B), to the right of the artery. Reversal of this indicates gut malrotation. The SMA supplies the small bowel from the mid point of the second part of the duodenum to the mid/distal transverse colon. The inferior mesenteric artery (IMA) supplies the remainder of the colon. The colon at the region of the splenic flexure is considered a watershed area in terms of vascularity and is a common site of ischaemia.

Case 15.14

A Right proximal humeral epiphyseal plate

B Right coracoid

C Spinous process of T1

D Right lower lobe pulmonary artery

E Right acromion

The scapula ossifies from at least seven different centres. A large proportion of the scapula ossifies in utero. The coracoid and acromion each have two ossification centres which begin to ossify between the 14th and 20th months of age. Ossification of the scapula is normally complete by 25 years of age. Ossification centres of the head, lesser tuberosity and greater tubercles of the humerus develop separately but fuse together to form the epiphysis. The proximal humeral epiphyseal plate is cone-shaped (with the apex pointing posteriorly, medially and superiorly) and usually fuses by the age of 22 years.

Case 15.15

A Body of testis

B Epididymis

C Vas deferens

D Mediastinum of testis

E Left renal vein

The mediastinum of the testis is a fibrous band through the mid body of the testis in which the vessels and nerves enter the gland. It is seen as a hyperechoic area (D) on ultrasound. The epididymis is seen posteriorly with the vas deferens coursing through it. The pampiniform plexus is the venous drainage of the testis. Each pampiniform plexus joins to form a testicular vein, of which the left drains into the left renal vein and the right directly into the IVC.

Case 15.16

A Foramen transversarium of the axis (C2)

B Subclavian artery

C Vertebral artery

D Carotid bifurcation

E Superior thyroid artery

The four major arteries on each side of the neck are:

1. **Common carotid artery** – bifurcates at the level of C4 vertebral body into its internal and external branches at the carotid bifurcation

2. **Internal carotid artery** – does not give off any branches in the neck

3. **External carotid artery** – eight branches are described, supplying the cervical organs, face, scalp and dura.

'Several Angry Ladies Fighting Over PMS' is a useful mnemonic for memorising:

Several – Superior thyroid artery

Angry – Ascending pharyngeal artery

Ladies – Lingual artery

Fighting – Facial artery

Over – Occipital artery

P – Posterior auricular artery

M – Maxillary artery

S – Superficial temporal artery

4. **Vertebral artery** – the first branch of the subclavian artery which travels through the foramina transversaria of the cervical vertebrae prior to entering the skull via foramen magnum.

Case 15.17

A Placenta

B Fetal brain

C Maternal bladder

D L3/4 intervertebral disc

E Third trimester

MRI is becoming more frequently used in pregnancy to determine possible pathology in both the fetus and the mother, without the inherent dangers of radiation exposure associated with CT. Placental position, fetal growth and gestational age, congenital anomalies and amniotic fluid appearances can all be readily visualised on MRI. In this image, the placenta lies anteriorly and well above the internal os, with the fetus in the normal cephalic presentation, a normal cord position and a normal amount of amniotic fluid.

Case 15.18

A Right pectineus muscle

B Right femoral head

C Right seminal vesicle

D Rectum

E Coccyx

The femoral canal is the space medial to the femoral vein and lateral to the lacunar ligament. The roof of the canal is the inguinal ligament and the floor is formed by the pectineus muscle.

The mnemonic **NAVY** may be used to remember the structures of the femoral canal, from lateral to medial:

Nerve, Artery, Vein, Y fronts.

Case 15.19

A Common hepatic artery

B Infrarenal aorta

C Right common iliac artery

D Left internal iliac artery

E Retroaortic left renal vein

The major aortic branches are depicted including coeliac axis, hepatic artery, splenic artery and iliac bifurcation. Note the dual left renal arteries and veins and also the retroaortic path of the left renal veins. Retroaortic left renal vein has a reported incidence of 1.8–2.4%.

Case 15.20

A Supraclinoid (intracranial) segment of the right internal carotid artery

B Left anterior cerebral artery

C M1 segment of the left middle cerebral artery

D Left posterior cerebral artery

E Absence of the left posterior communicating (P-com) artery

A complete circle of Willis (**Figure 15.1**) is seen in less than 50% of population. There are many potential anatomical variations, of which hypoplasia or absence of one of the P-com arteries is the most common (25–33% of cases).

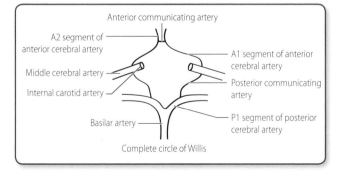

Figure 15.1 Schematic illustration of the complete circle of Willis.

Hypoplasia or absence of the A1 segment of the anterior cerebral artery is present in 10–20%.

Fetal origin of the posterior cerebral artery (PCA) with hypoplasia of the P1 segment (in which the PCA is supplied by the internal carotid artery via P-com) is present in 15–25%.

Index

A

Abdominal aorta
  course of left renal vein 420
  estimating lumbar vertebra level
  55
  IVC variations and 147
  MR angiogram 364
  pancreas and 302
  phrenic arteries 149
  sagittal midline view 272
  testicular artery 23
Abdominal CT 209
Abdominal wall 24, 244, 367, 453
  see also Diaphragm
Abducens nerve (CN VI) 52, 53
Abductor hallucis muscle 209
Abductor pollicis longus 150
Accessory fissures 392, 450, 451
Accessory nerve (CN XI) 28
Accessory ossicles of foot 425
Acetabulum 120, 152, 338, 422
Achilles tendon 54, 178
Acromioclavicular (AC) joint 144,
  211, 335
Acromion 144, 211, 455
Acromion process 176
Adductor hiatus 307
Adductor muscles 115, 149, 180, 181,
  184, 363, 394
Adrenal (suprarenal) glands 26, 149, 300
Alpha angle 152
Alveolar process, mandible 244
Amniotic cavity 182
Amniotic fluid 423, 456
Anal canal 149, 336
Anconeus muscle 426, 450
Angiography
  aortic arch 391
  internal carotid artery 82
  MR of mediastinum and neck 364
  pelvic vessels 396–7
  pulmonary artery 54, 301, 330
  vertebrobasilar circulation 146–7,
  241–2
Angularis incisura 176, 305
Ankle 121, 209, 365–6
  tendons 54, 365, 366, 392
Antecubital vein 180
Anterior cerebral artery (ACA) 273, 337,
  396, 457, 458
Anterior commissure 183
Anterior communicating artery (ACom)
  273, 337, 396, 457
Anterior cruciate ligament (ACL) 333
Anterior inferior cerebral artery (AICA)
  147

Anterior junctional lines 25
Anterior superior iliac spine (ASIS) 181
Anterior tibial artery 331, 332, 361
Anus 149, 336
Aorta
  abdominal *see* Abdominal aorta
  anatomic levels of structures 242
  aorto-pulmonary angle 52
  ascending 25, 116, 144, 422
  axial CTs 334
  bronchial arterial anatomy 184
  descending thoracic 177, 303, 334,
  392, 425
  infrarenal 457
  pelvic arterial tree 60
  pigtail catheter in distal 118
  portal vein and 86
  on T1-weighted axial sequence
  212
  testicular artery and 181
  see also Aortic arch
Aortic arch 54, 90, 176, 276
  aberrant right subclavian artery
  366, 453
  bovine 23–4
  common anatomical configuration
  144
  double (DAA) 274–5
  DSA angiography 391
  identifying asymptomatic right
  239
  identifying pulmonary trunk within
  393
  impression on oesophagus 27, 28,
  239
  'retro' spaces 306
  types of right-sided 177
Aortic sinuses 88, 151
Aortic valve 423, 451
Aortopulmonary angle/window 52,
  393
Appendix, vermiform 121, 239
Aqueous humour 335
Arachnoid mater 179, 238, 426
Arterial ligament 52, 393
Arthrography 304, 422
Arytenoid cartilages 183, 184
Atlantodental interval 335
Atlas (C1) 58–9
  arch of 56, 216, 334, 335
  atlantoaxial joint 150
  atlanto-occipital joint 305
Atria, cardiac
  apical 4-chamber echocardiogram
  148
  axial imaging 211

bronchial arterial anatomy 184
carina and 395
contrast swallow examinations 28
heart border 145–6, 395
high resolution CT scan 268
identification 332
as landmark 393
oblique coronal view 243
papillary muscle function 423
posterior wall of left 367
pulmonary angiography 54, 330
pulmonary venograms 54
'retro' spaces 306
right 423, 451
sagittal views 116
septal defects 27
Atrioventricular defects 27
Auditory canal
  external 28, 246, 302, 451
  internal 144, 151, 213
Auditory ossicles 144, 145, 246
Auricular artery 456
Avulsion injuries 55, 56, 243
Axilla, breast tissue 149
Axillary artery 85–6, 210, 334
Axillary lymph node 148
Axillary vein 26, 180, 426, 427
Axis (C2)
  atlantoaxial joint 150
  foramen transversarium 455
  odontoid process 29, 56, 58, 59,
  150, 333, 334
Azygo-oesophageal recess 83
Azygos lobe/fissure 52, 114, 118, 451
Azygos venous system 83, 114, 118,
  147, 242, 332, 392, 425

B

Barium enema examinations 121, 336
Basal vein of Rosenthal 305
Basilar artery (BA)
  cerebral veins and 305
  circle of Willis 396, 457
  formation 26
  as landmark 52, 53
  PCA as terminal branches 242
  vertebrobasilar circulation 146–7,
  241–2, 246, 361
  on view of oculomotor nerve 269
Basilar tip 146
Basilic vein 180, 426, 427
Basion 274
Benign prostatic hyperplasia 86
Biceps brachii muscle 84, 238, 272, 273
Biceps brachii tendon 336, 390, 391, 450

Biceps femoris muscle 115, 184, 185, 364, 394
Biceps femoris tendon 334
Biliary system 54–5, 118, 122, 214, 246, 450
Biparietal diameter 57, 182
Bladder see Urinary bladder
Bovine aortic arch 24
Bowel gas 59, 209, 215, 270
Brachial artery 214, 426
Brachial plexus 179, 304
Brachial vein 180, 426, 427
Brachialis muscle 453, 454
Brachiocephalic artery 23–4, 58, 144, 210, 334, 364, 391
Brachiocephalic veins 26, 91, 92, 144, 427
Brachioradialis muscle 426, 450
Brain 24
  cerebral envelope 178–9, 238, 426
  circle of Willis 396, 457
  coronal images 304
  corpus callosum 365, 420
  cranial nerves from 52
  CSF relationships 119
  fetal 456
  lobes and fissures 27, 362, 390
  motor cortex 390, 420
  neonates 214–15, 365
  pineal gland 115
  pituitary gland 24, 87
  septum pellucidum 27
  white matter tracts 420
Brainstem 52, 215, 238
Breast 148–9, 151, 275
Bregma 307
Broad ligament 117
Bronchial artery 184
Bronchus 22, 25
  arterial anatomy 184
  hilum 335
  impression on oesophagus 27, 28
  lateral segmental of middle lobe 365
  left main 276, 395
  lingular segments 240
  right main 421
  segmental architecture of lung 208
Bulbourethral gland 24, 25

C
Caecum 83, 121, 215
Calcaneum 60, 91, 121, 178, 245
Callosomarginal artery 273
Canine teeth 116
Capital femoral epiphysis 146, 215
Capitate bone 114, 182, 216, 268, 337, 360
Capitulum 302
  anterior humeral line 330
  articulation with radius 238, 273
  ossification centre 29, 119, 120, 182, 183, 362
  radiocapitellar line 330
Cardinal veins 92, 147, 303

Carina 52, 395, 453
Carotid artery
  carotid space 89, 427
  common 23–4, 209, 210, 242, 274, 334, 364, 391, 452, 456
  external 58, 337, 452, 455–6
  internal see Internal carotid artery
  right 88
  ultrasound examination 452
Carotid canal 28
Carotid space 89, 427
Carpal bones
  alignment 216, 268
  mnemonic for 114, 360
  orientation 82, 238
  ossification 337
Carpal tunnel 307
Caudate nucleus 214, 304
Cavernous sinuses 24
Cavum septum pellucidum (CSP) 27
Cavum septum pellucidum et vergae 27
Central sulcus (Rolandic fissure) 362, 390
Centrum semiovale 390
Cephalic vein 26, 180, 426, 427
Cerebellar arteries 146–7, 241, 269
Cerebellopontine angle (CPA) 52, 53
Cerebellum 181–2
  cerebellar vermis 181
  folia 25
  left hemisphere 361
  neonates 215, 365
  nodule of 181
  right hemisphere 276
Cerebral artery
  anterior 273, 337, 396, 457, 458
  left middle 331, 457
  posterior see Posterior cerebral arteries (PCA)
  right middle 24, 337
Cerebral veins 305
Cerebrospinal fluid (CSF) 119, 182, 238, 331, 420
Cerebrum, fetal 182
Cervical artery 58, 210
Cervical spine 180
  anterior tubercle of C5 246
  atlantoaxial joint 150
  atlantodental interval 335
  atlas (C1) 29, 56, 58–9, 150, 216, 305, 334, 335
  axis (C2) 56, 58, 59, 150, 455
    see also Odontoid process
  brachial plexus 304
  C5/6 intervertebral disc 58
  C7/T1 junction 216, 397
  craniocervical junction 29, 58–9, 274
  CT myelography 424
  dysphagia and 240
  exiting nerve roots 90, 361
  foramen transversarium 246
  inferior articular process of C4 216, 361
  odontoid process 29, 56, 58, 59, 150, 333, 334
  peg views 150

right lamina of C5 246
right transverse process of C5 300
right transverse process of C7 118
STIR MRI 272
trapezius muscle 276
uncinate process of C5 300
Cervix 58, 210, 211, 269
  of pregnant patient 336, 337
Children
  abdominal radiographs 274
  atlantodental interval 335
  bowel loop displacement 59
  cavum septum pellucidum 27
  cranial ultrasound 365
  fontanelles 307
  foot 60
  hypertrophic pyloric stenosis 122
  micturating cystourethrography 396
  ossification centres see Ossification centres
  skull fractures 421
  spinal cord visualisation 426
  ultrasound view of hip 152
Cingulate gyrus 365
Circle of Willis 396, 457
Circumflex arteries 85, 86, 271, 424, 451
Cisterna magna 181, 238
Cisterns
  interpeduncular 151, 238, 304
  prepontine 238
  quadrigeminal 119, 181, 238, 305
Clavicle 27, 179
  aberrant right subclavian artery and 366
  fetal 57
  lateral part 211
  left 144, 300
  right 239
  swimmer's view 397
  trapezius–deltoid differentiation 240
Clinoid process 366, 451
Clivus 302, 425
Coccyx 120, 183, 243, 336, 456
Cochlea 52, 145
Cochlear nerve 151, 213
Coeliac axis 271
  arises from the aorta 120, 422
  duodenal blood supply 176, 391
  main branches 85, 394
  portal vein–aorta relation 86
  sagittal midline view 272
Colic arteries 83, 303, 360
Collateral ligaments 333, 334
Colon 83
  ascending 83, 212, 239, 454
  descending 83, 85, 121, 215
  in double contrast 336
  inferior mesenteric artery 361
  presacral space 336
  rectum see Rectum
  sigmoid 82, 83, 121, 152, 210, 215, 243
  superior mesenteric artery 360, 454

transverse 24, 82, 83, 85, 122, 243
  visualised bones 121
Commissural tracts 420
Common femoral artery (CFA) 306
Communicating arteries 242, 273, 337, 396, 457
Conchae (turbinates), nasal 425
Confluence of venous sinuses 210
Conus, eye 25
Conus medullaris 53, 183, 454
Coracoid process of scapula
  left 335
  ligaments attaching to 176
  muscles attaching to 273, 305, 306
  orientation by 57, 144, 211
  ossification centres 455
  right 145, 454
  swimmer's view 397
Cornea 335
Coronal imaging 239
Coronal suture 307, 421
Coronary artery 87, 88, 116, 151, 268, 271, 451
Coronoid fossa of humerus 273, 362
Coronoid process
  mandible 56, 244, 333
  ulna 238, 302, 453, 454
Corpus callosum 365, 420
Corpus cavernosum 331, 367, 427
Corpus spongiosum 367, 427
Corticobulbar pathway 420
Corticospinal pathway 420
Costo-bronchial trunk 366
Costocervical trunk 58, 274, 334, 366
Costotransverse joint 300, 306
Costovertebral joint 151, 300, 305, 306
Couinaud classification 214, 397–8
Cowper's gland 24, 25
Cranial nerves see Abducens nerve (CN VI); Accessory nerve (CN XI); Facial nerve (CN VII); Glossopharyngeal nerve (CN IX); Hypoglossal nerve (CN XII); Oculomotor nerve (CN III); Trigeminal nerve (CN V); Vagus nerve (CN X); Vestibulocochlear nerve (CN VIII)
Cranial ultrasound, neonates 365
Craniocervical junction 29, 58–9, 274
Craniosynostosis 421
Cricoid cartilage 183, 209, 242
CRITOL 29, 120, 183
Cruciate ligaments 333
CT myelography 53, 424
CT urography 53
Cuboid bone 59, 60, 91, 178, 245, 392
Cuneiform bones 26, 54, 60, 91, 121, 178, 392
Cystic duct 54, 55, 118
Cystic fibrosis 184
Cystourethrography, micturating 396

D

Deltoid ligament 209
Deltoid muscle 240, 272, 273, 390, 391
Dens see Odontoid process (peg)
Dental orthopantomograms (OPGs) 116

Descending colon 83, 85, 121, 215
Diaphragm
  abdominal wall division 24
  crura of 178
  fetal 57
  hiatuses 28
  left hemidiaphragm 152, 367, 452
  parasagittal views 452
  right hemidiaphragm 27, 118, 178
Diencephalon 115
Digital subtraction angiography (DSA)
  aortic arch 391
  internal carotid artery 82
  vertebrobasilar circulation 146–7, 241–2
Diverticulum of Kommerell 150, 453
Double aortic arch (DAA) 274–5
Ductus venosus 337
Duodenojejunal junction 176, 239, 305
Duodenum 85, 118, 176, 215
  blood supply 176, 391, 394
  distal 390
  duodenal cap 305
  four parts of 391
  nutcracker syndrome 272
Dura mater 178, 179, 426
Dural layer 178
Dural sinuses 210

E

Ear 28, 52, 144–5, 151, 213, 245–6, 302, 451
Elbow
  brachial artery 214
  lateral radiograph 330
  ossification centres 29, 119–20, 182, 183, 362
  sagittal MRI of medial 453–4
Embryological development
  chambers of heart 332
  double aortic arch 275
  gastrointestinal tract 85
  inferior vena cava 367
  testes 181
  venous system 92, 303
Endometrium 115, 210, 211, 239, 269, 301, 393
Epididymis 181, 455
Epigastric vessels 59, 210, 277
Epiglottis 117, 183, 212, 335
Epitympanum 245, 246
Erector spinae muscles 24, 55, 89, 244, 272, 334, 338, 454
Ethmoid infundibulum 176, 177
Ethmoid ostium 425
Extensor carpi radialis 150, 303
Extensor carpi ulnaris 150, 303
Extensor digiti minimi 150, 303
Extensor digitorum 150, 303
Extensor indicis 150
Extensor pollicis 150
External auditory canal/meatus 28, 246, 302, 451
External carotid artery (ECA) 58, 337, 452, 455–6

External oblique muscles 244, 453
Extradural space 178
Extraocular muscles 25
Eye 25, 335

F

Facet joints 120, 121, 335, 360, 361
Facial artery 456
Facial bones 243–4
  fracture assessment 333
  lateral views 366
  muscular and ligamentous attachments 56
  zygomatic arch 28, 243
  see also Frontal bone; Mandible; Maxilla; Nasal bone
Facial nerve (CN VII) 52, 89, 145, 151, 213
Falciform ligament 337
Fallopian tubes 58, 117
Falx cerebri 27, 119, 178, 390
Fat
  intra-abdominal 209
  pericardial 332, 425
  retro-orbital 25
Fat pad
  elbow joint 362
  infrapatellar 22, 271
Femoral arteries 60, 306–7, 424
Femoral canal 456–7
Femoral vein 54, 86, 367
Femur
  capital femoral epiphysis 146, 215, 396
  distal diaphysis 22
  fluoroscopic arthrography 304
  fovea of head of 91, 277
  frontal knee radiograph 452
  greater trochanter 59, 146, 215, 245, 397, 421
  head of left 420
  head of right 456
  identifying superior acetabulum 338
  intercondylar notch 451
  lateral condyle 300, 301, 451
  medial condyle 333, 334, 362
  muscle/tendon attachments 55, 91, 146, 181, 184, 421
  pectineus muscle 28
  right 180, 424
Fetal imaging 336–7
  fontanelles 307
  gestational age assessment 57, 182, 424, 456
  heart scans 27
  MRI 423–4, 456
  see also Embryological development
Fibula
  distal 178, 245, 392
  frontal knee radiograph 452
  head of 271, 301, 333, 334, 451
  tibiofibular joint 22, 271
  tibiofibular syndesmosis 365, 366
Filum terminale 53, 183, 454
Finger(s) 82, 182

Flexor carpi radialis 303
Flexor carpi ulnaris 303
Flexor digitorum longus 26, 366
Flexor digitorum profundus 307
Flexor digitorum superficialis 216,
303, 307
Flexor hallucis brevis 26
Flexor hallucis longus 54, 366
Flexor pollicis longus 307
Flexor retinaculum 307
Flexor tendon, common 302, 303
Fluoroscopic arthrography 304, 422
Fluoroscopic lumbar myelography 53
Folia of cerebellum 25
Fontanelles 307
Foot
　accessory ossicles 425
　ankle tendon insertion 54, 121
　fundamental anatomy 26, 178, 392
　hallucal sesamoid bones 91
　oblique radiograph of child's
　59–60
　orientation tips 121
　ossification centres 60, 245
Foramen magnum 243, 274, 275, 276
Foramen ovale 302
Foramen rotundum 84, 395
Foramen spinosum 302
Foramina transversaria 246, 424
Fornix, cerebral 114, 420
Frog leg pelvic radiograph 215
Frontal bone, fetal 57
Frontal lobe 362
Frontal recess 177
Frontal sinus 213
Frontozygomatic suture 176, 394

G
Galen, great vein of 305
Gallbladder 54, 118, 145, 334, 363, 422
Gas in bowel 59, 209, 215, 270
Gastric anatomy see Stomach
Gastric artery 422
Gastroduodenal artery 176, 394, 422
Gastroepiploic artery 394
Gastrointestinal tract development 85
Gastro-oesophageal junction 152, 242
Genioglossus muscle 148, 392, 393
Genu of corpus callosum 420
Gerbode defect 27
Glenohumeral joint 83, 211, 391
Glenoid fossa of temporal bone 423
Glenoid of scapula 57, 83, 211, 240, 336
Glossopharyngeal nerve (CN IX) 28
Gluteal arteries 213, 214, 396, 397
Gluteal muscles 151, 245, 304, 397
　gluteus maximus 59, 146, 149, 245,
　367, 422
　gluteus medius 26, 245, 363, 421
　gluteus minimus 245, 363, 367,
　396, 421
Gonadal vein 153
Gracilis muscle 28, 115, 146, 180,
184, 394
Great vein of Galen 305
Gut malrotation 88, 454
Guyon's canal 307

Gyri 362, 390
　cingulate 365
　parahippocampal 304

H
Habenula 115
Hamate bone 82, 114, 337
Hamstring muscles 56, 115, 185, 394
Hand 82, 182, 216, 307, 337, 360
Haustra 336
Heart atria see Atria, cardiac
Heart border silhouettes 145–6, 240,
365, 395
Heart chambers see Atria, cardiac;
Ventricles, cardiac
Heart disease, congenital 275
Heart scans, fetal 27
Hepatic artery 214, 246, 363, 394, 398,
422, 457
Hepatic duct, common 54, 55, 118,
450
Hepatic veins 23, 53, 120, 145, 152,
242, 363, 398
Herniograms 277
Heterotaxy syndromes 303
Hiatus hernias 83
Hiatus semilunaris (HS) 177
Hilar point 335
Hilum 335, 367
Hip
　fluoroscopic arthrography 304,
　422
　left 179
　MR imaging 422
　ossification centre 396
　ultrasound of infant 152
Hippocampus 304
Hoffa's fat pad 22, 271
Horizontal fissure 367
Humerus
　anterior humeral line 330
　bicipital groove 336, 391
　capitulum see Capitulum
　coronoid fossa 273, 362
　distal 302
　see also Capitulum; Lateral epicon-
　dyle; Medial epicondyle; Trochlea
　glenohumeral joint 83, 211, 391
　head of 144, 240, 336, 397
　key osseous anatomy of distal 273
　lateral epicondyle 29, 120, 183,
　273, 303
　on lateral radiograph of elbow 330
　medial epicondyle 29, 119, 120,
　183, 273, 303
　neck of right 85
　nutrient artery 214
　ossification centres 29, 83, 119,
　120, 183, 362, 455
　proximal 390, 391
　proximal epiphyseal plate 454, 455
　radiocapitellar line 330
　rotator cuff attachments 57, 84
　sagittal MRI of elbow 453–4
　swimmer's view 397
　trochlea 29, 119, 120, 183, 273,
　302, 330, 453

Hydrocoeles 181
Hyoid bone 239, 270, 335, 364, 424
Hypertrophic pyloric stenosis 122
Hypoglossal canals 275, 276
Hypoglossal nerve (CN XII) 275, 276
Hypoglossus muscle 148
Hypopharynx 117, 212, 364, 365
Hypophyseal fossa 451
Hypothalamus 87, 115
　neonates 215
Hysterosalpingography 58, 117

I
Ileocaecal valve 239
Ileocolic branch of SMA 83, 303, 360,
454
Ileum 121
Iliac arteries 60, 118, 152, 213, 214, 360
　common femoral artery 306, 424
　left common 361
　left external 396
　left internal 396, 457
　right common 422, 457
　umbilical arterial catheters 274
　uterine arteries from 393
Iliac veins 54, 59, 152
Iliacus muscle
　iliopsoas formation 55
　left 367
　MR imaging of the hip 422
　origins 91, 363
　parts of abdominal wall 24
　right 53, 245, 301
Iliolumbar artery 213, 214
Iliopectineal line 23, 116, 277
Iliopsoas bursa 304
Iliopsoas muscle 55, 146, 363
Iliopsoas tendon 421, 422
Iliotibial band/tract 28, 115, 146, 334
Ilium 152
　crest 59, 120, 363
　MR imaging of the hip 422
　osseous acetabulum 338
　right 396
　sacroiliac joint 53, 117, 209, 245,
　304, 390
　spine 55, 180, 181, 243
　triradiate cartilage 215
　tubercle 28
　wing 59
　see also Sacroiliac joint
Incisor teeth 116, 150
Incisura angularis 176, 305
Incudomalleolar joint 144, 145
Incus 145, 246
Infants see Children
Inferior epigastric vessels 59
Inferior mesenteric artery (IMA) 83, 85,
122, 360, 361
Inferior thyroid artery 210
Inferior vena cava (IVC) 23, 53, 88
　embryology 367
　flow artefacts 300
　hepatic veins converging on 145,
　363
　intrahepatic 23, 26
　landmark in sagittal views 122

liver segment I 214, 399
lumbar vertebra level estimation 55
    main tributaries 152–3
    maternal 423
    portal vein–common hepatic duct and 450
    pulmonary angiography 54
    testicular vein draining to 181
    variations 120, 147, 212
Infrapatellar (Hoffa's) fat pad 22, 271
Infraspinatus muscle 57, 83, 84, 144, 305, 306, 336
Infundibulum
    ethmoid 176, 177
    pituitary 87
Inguinal hernias 277
Inguinal ligaments 244
Innominate artery see Brachiocephalic artery
Insular cortex 215
Intercostal nerve 334
Intercostal vessels 58, 184, 334
Interhemispheric fissure 27, 390
Internal auditory canal/meatus (IAM) 144, 151, 213
Internal carotid artery (ICA)
    branches 273, 456
    carotid canal 28
    cavernous portion 24, 82, 337
    left 26
    petrous portion 396
    supraclinoid segment 457
    ultrasound examination 452
Internal oblique muscles 244, 361, 452, 453
Internal thoracic artery 210, 268, 274, 366, 391
Interosseous artery 214
Interpeduncular cisterns 151, 238, 304
Interphalangeal joints 392
Interventricular septum 27, 56, 148, 211, 332
Intervertebral discs 147, 301
    assessing nerve root compression 55
    C5/C6 58
    CT myelography 424
    fetal MRI 456
    fluoroscopic lumbar myelography 53
    L4/L5 28
    posterior longitudinal ligament 29
Intravenous urography (IVU) 87
Ischioanal fossae 149, 367
Ischium
    ischial ramus 55
    ischial spine 55, 243, 277
    ischial tuberosity 394
    osseous acetabulum 338
    right 149, 274
    triradiate cartilage 215

J
Jejunal branch of SMA 303, 360, 422, 454

Jejunum 176, 390
    duodenojejunal junction 176, 239, 305
Jugular foramen 28
Jugular veins 28
    axial STIR MRI 272
    carotid space 89
    internal 144, 183, 208, 210, 242, 427
Junction lines 25

K
Kidney 178
    left 454
    left-sided varicocoeles 181
    maternal 423
    pelviureteric junction 87
    suprarenal (adrenal) glands 26
    on T1-weighted axial sequence 212
    transplantation 118
    ultrasound imaging 332
    urography 53, 87
Knee
    articular cartilage of patella 395
    cruciate ligaments 395
    frontal radiograph 452
    infrapatellar fat pad 22, 271
    medial meniscus 333, 334
    patellar tendon 22, 395
    quadriceps tendon 364
    sagittal images 300, 301
Kommerell, diverticulum of 150, 453

L
Labrum
    acetabular 152, 422
    anterior glenoid 83, 336
Labyrinth, inner ear 145
Lambdoid suture 307, 421
Laryngeal nerve 52, 393
Laryngopharynx see Hypopharynx
Larynx
    cartilages 183, 209, 242, 246, 427
    piriform fossae 212, 364
    vocal cords 183
Lateral collateral ligament 333, 334
Lateral epicondyle 29, 120, 183, 273, 303
Lateral sulcus (sylvian fissure) 119, 362
Latissimus dorsi muscle 91, 242
Lens, eye 25, 335
Lentiform nucleus 215, 304
Levator ani muscles 149, 240, 241
Levator palpebrae superioris 25
Ligamentum arteriosum 52, 393
Ligamentum flavum 29
Ligamentum teres 91
Limbic system 304
Lingual artery 456
Lingula of lung 240, 392, 451
Lip, lower 366
Lister's tubercle 150
Liver 59
    Couinaud classification 214, 397–8
    fetal 57

left lobe 86, 270, 271, 420
    right lobe 24, 209, 246, 276, 332
    ultrasound for hypertrophic pyloric stenosis 122
    venous system 23, 86, 214, 215, 363
Longissimus capitis muscle 56
Longitudinal ligament, posterior 29
Lumbar artery 118
Lumbar myelography 53
Lumbar spine
    CT myelography 424
    estimating level of 55
    exiting nerve root levels 55, 90
    facet joint L3/L4 120
    fetal MRI 456
    fluorescent lumbar myelography 53
    L4 26
    L4 superior articular process 53
    L4/L5 intervertebral disc 28, 90
    L5 nerve root 53
    left L4 nerve root 89, 90
    left pars interarticularis of L1 89
    left pedicle of L1 89
    right L5 transverse process 176
    right pedicle of L2 209
    right transverse process of L3 55
    superior articular process of L5 120
    vertebral body of L5 331, 336
Lumbar veins 153
Lunate bone 114, 214, 216, 268
Lung 22, 25, 52
    accessory fissures 392, 450, 451
    azygos lobe/fissure 52, 114, 118, 451
    bronchial arterial anatomy 184
    heart borders and 145, 240, 365, 395
    hilum 335, 367
    horizontal fissure 367
    left minor fissure 451
    left paraspinal line 85
    lingula 240, 392, 451
    lower lobe of right 334, 455
    middle lobe 392, 421
    oblique fissure 25, 240, 365, 367, 392, 450
    segmental architecture 208, 240, 365, 421
Lymph nodes
    azygo-oesophageal recess 83
    mammograms 148, 149
    mediastinal 52
    neck spaces 89
Lymphatic drainage, testes 181

M
Malleolus 209, 331, 365, 366, 392
Malleus 145, 245, 246
Mamillary body 87, 114
Mammary artery see Internal thoracic artery
Mammograms 148–9
Mandible
    alveolar process 244
    angle of 212, 244
    body of left hemimandible 150

body of 243, 392
condylar process 56, 216, 239, 244, 275, 423
coronoid process 56, 244, 333
genioglossus muscle 148
left ramus 243
masticator space 89
orthopantomograms 116
retromolar trigone 180
structures of 244
temporomandibular joint 56, 116, 423
Manubriosternal joint 149
Manubrium of malleus 245
Massa intermedia 114
Masseter muscle 88, 180
Masticator space 89
Mastoid air cells 243, 331
Mastoid bone 423
mastoid process 56
Maxilla
antrum 302
orthopantomograms 116
palatine process 270
Maxillary artery 58, 89, 456
Maxillary sinus 176–7, 212
Medial epicondyle 29, 119, 120, 183, 273, 303
Median nerve 307
Mediastinal pathologies
left paraspinal line 85
lymph node enlargement 52
Medulla oblongata 275
Meningeal artery 423
Meniscus 300, 301, 333, 334, 452
Mesenteric artery
inferior 83, 85, 122, 360, 361
superior see Superior mesenteric artery (SMA)
Mesenteric vein 215, 270
Metacarpals 82, 182, 216, 238, 337
Metatarsals 54, 121, 178, 245, 392
Metatarsophalangeal joint 26
Micturating cystourethrography 396
Midbrain colliculi 119
Midgut malrotation 88, 454
Mitral valve 27, 243, 268, 330, 423
Molar teeth 116, 180, 270
Motor cortex 390, 420
Mouth
floor of 392–3
teeth see Teeth
tongue muscles 56, 148, 393
vestibule 270
MRI
arthrography 304, 422
coronal 239
fetal 423–4, 456
flowing blood 367
signal near articulations 301
STIR 272
Myelography 53, 424
Mylohyoid muscle 392–3
Myometrium 115, 393

N
Nasal bone 28, 366
Nasal cavity 425

Nasal septum 116
Nasogastric tubes 59, 149, 274
Nasopharynx 117, 212, 366
Navicular bone 26, 178, 245, 425
Navicular fossa 25, 179
Neck
axial anatomy 180
spaces 88, 89, 117
structures at level VI 209
vascular anatomy 144, 455–6
Neonates
abdominal radiographs 274
brain 214–5, 365
cavum septum pellucidum 27
cranial ultrasound 365
displacement of bowel loops 59
fontanelles 307
spinal cord visualisation 426
Neurocentral joint of Luschka 300
Nipple 148, 275
Nuchal thickness 182
Nutcracker syndrome 272

O
Oblique fissure 25, 240, 365, 367, 392, 450
Oblique muscles
abdominal wall 244, 361, 452, 453
extraocular 25
Obstetric anaesthesia 243
Obstetric haemorrhage 393
Obturator externus muscle 421
Obturator foramen 23, 215, 396
Obturator internus muscle 28, 146, 240, 241, 393, 421
Obturator nerve 363
Occipital artery 456
Occipital bone 82, 334
fetal 57, 307
foramen magnum 243, 274, 275, 276
hypoglossal canal 275, 276
Occipital lobe 362, 365
Occipital sinus 210
Occipitomastoid suture 275, 421
Oculomotor nerve (CN III) 24, 269
Odontoid process (peg) 29, 56, 58, 59, 150, 333, 334
Oesophagus 28, 116, 177
aberrant left subclavian artery 239
aberrant right subclavian artery 150
anatomical levels 242
azygo-oesophageal recess 83
distal 242
double aortic arch 274–5
fluid in 151
persistent left SVC 303
pharynx and 212, 239, 240
Olecranon 29, 119, 120, 183, 330, 362, 426, 453–4
Ophthalmic artery 82
Opisthion 274
Optic canal 84
Optic chiasm 87, 330
Optic nerve 25
Optic sheath 335
Orbit 25, 335, 395

Orbital fissure, superior 84, 395
Oropharynx 88, 117, 180, 212, 239, 365, 392
Orthopantomograms (OPGs) 116
Os trigonum 425
Ossicles
accessory of foot 425
auditory 144, 145, 246
Ossification centres
elbow 29, 119–20, 182–3, 362
foot 60, 245
hand and wrist 82, 337
left femoral capital epiphysis 396
scapula 455
thumb 182
Osteomeatal complex 176–7, 425
Ovaries 301, 338

P
Paediatric anatomy see Children
Palate (hard) 116, 150
Palate (soft) 366
Palatine process of maxilla 270
Palatine tonsils 117
Palmaris longus 303
Pampiniform plexus 23, 181, 455
Pancreas 271, 300, 302
Pancreatic duct 118
Pancreaticoduodenal arteries 176, 391
Papillary muscles 56, 243, 268, 423
Parahippocampal gyrus 304
Parapharyngeal space 88, 89
Paraspinal line, left 85
Parietal bones 57, 182, 307
Parietal lobe 362
Parieto-occipital fissure 362
Parotid gland 58, 88, 89, 117, 180, 270
Parotid space 89
Pars interarticularis 120, 121
Patella 22, 271, 364, 395, 451
Patellar tendon 22, 271
Pectineus muscle 28, 394, 456
Pectoralis muscles 90, 148, 149
coracoid process and 272, 273, 306
MRI of breast 275
Pelvic bones
frog leg radiograph 215
muscular/tendinous attachments 55–6, 91, 146, 243, 363
osseous acetabulum 338
Pelvis
arterial tree 60
axial CT angiogram of male 396–7
axial T2-weighted MRI of male 86–7
bones see Pelvic bones
broad ligament 117
kidney transplantation 118
peritoneal reflections in 277
sagittal views through 211
transabdominal ultrasound of female 393
Pelviureteric junction 87
Penis 367
penile urethra 24, 179
Percutaneous transhepatic cholangiography (PTC) 55
Pericallosal artery 273, 305, 337

Pericardial effusion 148
Pericardial fluid traces 425
Perineal body 241
Peritoneal reflections 277
Peritoneum 85, 122
Peroneal artery 331, 332, 361
Peroneal tendons 54, 365, 366, 392
Pes anserine 181
Petrous temporal bone 28, 145
Phalanges 26, 59, 82, 182, 245, 360, 392
Pharyngeal artery 452, 456
Pharyngeal mucosal space 89, 117
Pharynx 117, 212
    hypopharynx 117, 212, 364, 365
    nasopharynx 117, 212, 366
    oropharynx 88, 117, 180, 212, 239, 365, 392
    retropharyngeal soft tissues 364
    spaces of neck 89, 117
Phrenic arteries 149, 210
Phrenic nerve 179
Phrenic veins 152
Pia mater 179, 183, 238, 426, 454
Pineal gland 115
Pinna 245, 451
Piriform fossae 212, 364
Piriformis muscle 59, 243, 396, 397
Pisiform bone 82, 114, 238, 337
Pituitary fossa 451
Pituitary gland 24, 87
Placenta 336, 337, 423, 456
Plantar fascia 425
Pneumoperitoneum 85
Pons 52, 331
Popliteal artery 307, 331, 332, 361, 364
Popliteal vein 364
Popliteus muscle 271
Portal venous system
    aorta–coeliac axis and 86
    classic view 246
    Couinaud classification of liver 214, 398
    formation 88, 270, 363
    gallbladder and 145
    IVC-common hepatic duct relation 450
    right portal vein 23, 122
    venous confluence 215, 300, 302, 420
Postcentral gyrus 362, 390
Posterior auricular artery 456
Posterior cerebral arteries (PCA)
    circle of Willis 396, 457
    fetal origin 458
    left 269
    right 304, 396
    vertebrobasilar circulation 146–7, 241–2
Posterior communicating artery 242, 337, 396, 457
Posterior cruciate ligament (PCL) 333
Posterior descending artery 87
Posterior internal iliac artery 213, 214
Posterior tibial artery 331, 332, 361
Precentral gyrus 362, 390
Pregnancy
    fetal heart scans 27
    fetal MRI 423, 456

gestational age assessment 57, 182, 424, 456
    obstetric anaesthesia 243
    obstetric haemorrhage 393
    parasagittal MRI 336–7
    see also Embryological develop-
    ment
Pre-molar teeth 116
Prepontine cisterns 238
Profunda brachii 214
Profunda femoris artery (PFA) 60, 306, 424
Pronator teres 303, 450
Prostate gland 86–7, 240, 241
Prostatic urethra 25, 179, 241, 331
Psoas muscles
    iliopsoas tendon 422
    insertion of psoas major 146
    left psoas major 24, 55, 87, 209, 367
    origin of psoas major 146
    right psoas major 53, 91, 212, 453
Pterygoid muscles 117
Pterygoid plates 84, 85
Pterygopalatine fossa 84
Pubic bones
    fluoroscopic arthrography 304
    muscle origins 28, 149, 394
    osseous acetabulum 338
    pubic ramus 55, 58, 146, 304, 336, 367
    symphysis pubis 23, 210, 331, 393, 394
    triradiate cartilage 215
Puborectalis muscle 149
Pudendal nerve blocks 243
Pulmonary artery 53–4, 116, 144, 330
    aorto-pulmonary angle 52
    coronary artery and 451
    delayed angiographic run 301
    hilar point 335
    identifying 393
    left lower lobe 176
    right 425
    right lower lobe 239, 335, 455
Pulmonary veins 151, 211, 240, 301, 335
Pulmonary venograms 54
Pylorus 122, 176, 390

Q

Quadratus femoris muscle 149
Quadratus lumborum muscle 24, 55
Quadriceps muscles 115, 181, 184, 364
Quadriceps tendon 22, 300, 364
Quadrigeminal cisterns 119, 181, 238, 305
Quadrigeminal (tectal) plate 115

R

Radial artery 214
Radio-ulnar joint 114
Radius
    distal 216
    distal epiphysis 337
    head of 29, 119, 120, 183, 273, 362, 426

key structures of forearm 450
Lister's tubercle 150
ossification centre 119, 120, 182, 183, 362
    proximal diaphysis 302
radio-ulnar joint 114
radiocapitellar line 330
radiolunate line 268
Rectal artery, superior 122
Recti muscles, extraocular 25
Rectum 59, 82, 331, 456
    axial T2-weighted MRI 86
    barium enema examinations 121
    divisions of the colon 83
    in double contrast 336
    gas filled 60
    presacral space 336
Rectus abdominis muscle 24, 59, 244, 245
Rectus femoris muscle 55, 115, 181, 243, 363, 364, 394
Renal artery 91, 149, 367, 422
Renal vein 120
    course of 420
    left IVC draining to 147
    retroaortic left 457
    superior mesenteric artery and 153, 272
    testicular vein draining to 23, 181, 455
    tributary of IVC 152
Retrograde urethrography 25
Retromolar trigone 180
Retropharyngeal space 89
Retropubic venous plexus 86, 87
Ribs 209, 239, 272
    costocervical trunk 58, 274, 334, 366
    costotransverse joint 300, 306
    costovertebral joint 151, 300, 305, 306
    fetal 57
    intercostal vessels 334
Right coronary artery (RCA) 87, 88, 116, 151
Rolandic fissure (central sulcus) 362, 390
Rosenthal, basal vein of 305
Rotator cuff 57, 83–4, 240
Round ligament see Ligamentum teres

S

Sacral artery, lateral 213, 214
Sacroiliac joint 53, 117, 178, 209, 245, 304, 390, 420
Sacrospinous ligament 243
Sacrotuberous ligament 243
Sacrum 116
    left alum 53, 338
    presacral space 336
    sacrospinous ligament 243
    see also Sacroiliac joint
Sagittal imaging 239
Sagittal sinuses 27, 178, 210, 305
Sagittal suture 307
Salivary glands 270
    parotid see Parotid gland

Sartorius muscle 55, 115, 181, 184, 243, 363, 364, 394, 427
Scalene muscles 179, 305
Scaphoid bone 114, 268
Scapholunate ligament 360
Scapula 57, 83–4
  body of 390
  coracoid process see Coracoid process of scapula
  glenoid of 57, 83, 211, 240, 336
  lateral view 144
  left 151
  ligament attachments 176
  muscle attachments 272, 305, 306, 336, 391
  ossification 455
  right 114, 421
  swimmer's view 397
Sciatic foramen 243, 397
Sciatic nerve 59, 115
Scrotum 181
Scutum 245, 246
Sella turcica 451
Semicircular canals 145
Semimembranosus muscle 115, 185, 394
Seminal vesicles 456
Semitendinosus muscle 180, 185, 394
Septal defects 27, 332
Septum pellucidum 27
Serratus anterior muscle 425
Sesamoid bones 26, 91, 238
Short tau inversion recovery (STIR) MRI 272
Shoulder 57, 83–4, 144, 211, 240, 391
Sialography 270
Sigmoid colon 82, 83, 121, 152, 210, 215, 243, 336
Sinoatrial node artery 87, 88
Skull
  bony processes 56
    see also Odontoid process
  craniocervical junction 29, 58–9, 274
  extradural space 178, 179
  fetal age assessment 57, 182
  fissures and foramina 28, 84, 243, 274, 275, 276, 302, 394–5
  infant 421
  parietal bones 57, 182, 307
  sutures 176, 275, 307, 394, 421
  wormian bone 307, 421
    see also Mandible
Spermatic cord 427
Sphenoid bone 84–5, 302, 394, 395, 451
Sphenoid sinuses 24, 84, 85, 117, 425
Spinal arteries 184
Spinal cord
  cardiac chambers on axial view 211
  cardiac chambers on coronal view 243
  cervical 180
  conus medullaris 53, 183, 454
  cranial nerves arising from 52
  descending pathways 420

filum terminale 53, 183, 454
fluoroscopic lumbar myelography 53
  motor cortex 390
  neonates 426
  spinal artery embolisation 184
  STIR MRI 272
  on view of liver 214
Spinal dysraphism 183, 454
Spinal nerve roots 53, 55, 89, 90, 361, 424
Spine see Cervical spine; Lumbar spine; Thoracic spine
Spinous processes 118, 121, 145, 176, 183, 276, 426, 455
Spleen 120, 178
Splenic artery 53, 88, 214, 422
Splenic vein 88, 215, 270, 300, 302, 363
Splenius capitis muscle 56
Spondylolisthesis 121
Spondylolysis 121
Stapes 145, 246
Stensen, duct of 270
Sternoclavicular joint 177, 422
Sternocleidomastoid muscle 56, 179, 208, 209, 392, 424, 427, 452
Sternum 90, 306
  STIR MRI 272
Stomach 120, 390
  angular notch 305
  in diaphragmatic assessment 452
  fundus 59, 83, 178, 239, 335
  gas in 209, 270
  gastroepiploic artery 394
  lesser curve 334, 390
  lumen 26
  milk curd in 122
  nomenclature 390
  pylorus 122, 176, 390
  wall thickness 300
Straight sinus 210, 305
Styloglossus muscle 56, 148
Stylohyoid muscle 56
Styloid process
  temporal bone 56
  ulna 82, 114
Stylopharyngeus muscle 56
Subarachnoid cisterns see Cisterns
Subarachnoid space 178, 179, 426, 454
Subclavian artery 58, 85, 144, 179, 455
  aberrant left 239
  aberrant right 149, 150, 177, 366, 391, 453
  mnemonic for branches of 210
  MR angiogram 364
  right 274, 450
Subclavian vein 26, 144, 179, 427, 450
Subdural space 179
Sublingual gland 270
Sublingual space 393
Submandibular gland 270
Submandibular space 393
Subscapular artery 86
Subscapularis muscle 57, 83, 84, 305, 306, 390, 391
Sulci, cortical 119, 362, 390
Superficial femoral artery (SFA) 306–7, 424

Superficial temporal artery 456
Superior cerebellar artery (SCA) 146, 147, 241, 269
Superior epigastric vessels 210
Superior glenoid tubercle 83, 84
Superior mesenteric artery (SMA) 85, 86, 152
  branches 83, 303, 360, 454
  duodenal blood supply 391
  formation 120
  jejunal branch 303, 360, 422
  left renal vein and 153, 420
  midgut malrotation 88
  nutcracker syndrome 272
  sagittal midline view 272
  superior mesenteric vein and 270
Superior mesenteric vein 215, 270, 363, 454
Superior rectal artery 122
Superior rectus muscle 25
Superior sagittal sinus 27, 178, 210
Superior vena cava (SVC) 26, 91, 92, 144, 177, 303, 365, 425
Supinator muscle 450
Suprarenal (adrenal) glands 26, 149, 300
Suprarenal artery 149
Suprarenal vein 152
Suprascapular artery 210
Suprasellar cistern 238, 330, 396
Supraspinatus muscle 57, 84, 144, 240, 306
Sutures of skull 176, 275, 307, 394, 421
Swimmer's view 397
Sylvian fissure (lateral sulcus) 119, 362
Symphysis pubis 23, 210, 331, 393, 394

T
Taeniae coli 336
Talonavicular joint 121
Talus 59, 60, 91, 121, 178, 209, 245, 365, 424, 425
Tarsal bones 26, 54, 59–60, 91, 121, 178, 245, 392
Tarsometatarsal joint 178
Tectal (quadrigeminal) plate 115
Tectorial membrane 29
Teeth 116, 150, 180, 270
Temporal artery 58, 456
Temporal bone
  glenoid fossa 423
  mastoid portion 56, 423
  petrous portion 28, 145
  styloid process 56
Temporal lobe 304, 362
Temporalis muscle 56
Temporomandibular joint (TMJ) 56, 116, 423
Temporo-occipital incisure 362
Temporosquamal suture 421
Tensor fascia lata muscle 115, 146, 184
Teres major muscle 214
Teres minor muscle 57, 84
Testes 23, 181, 427, 455
Testicular artery 23, 181
Testicular vein 23, 455

Thalamus 115
Thecal sac 420, 424
Thigh
    muscles 28, 115, 181, 184–5, 394
    superficial femoral artery 307
Thoracic arteries 85, 86
    internal thoracic artery 210, 268,
    274, 366, 391
Thoracic spinal cord 243
Thoracic spine
    body of T10 242
    brachial plexus 304
    C7/T1 junction 216, 397
    CT myelography 424
    exiting nerve roots 90, 361
    oesophageal traverse of diaphragm
    28
    right pedicle of T5 52
    right pedicle of T7 118
    right transverse process of T2 83
    right transverse process of T12 334
    spinous process of T1 455
    spinous process of T2 118, 145,
    176
    trapezius muscle 276
    winking owl sign 118
Thoracoacromial artery 86
3D SPACE 52
Thumb 82, 182, 238, 360
Thymus 83
Thyrocervical trunk 210
Thyroid artery 210, 455, 456
Thyroid cartilage 183, 209, 242, 246,
    427
Thyroid gland 242, 427
Thyroid isthmus 209
Tibia
    frontal knee radiograph 452
    iliotibial band/tract 28, 115, 146,
    334
    lateral condyle 300, 301
    medial prominence of spine of 451
    proximal tibiofibular joint 22, 271
    tibiofibular syndesmosis 365, 366
    tuberosity 271
Tibial arteries 54, 331, 332, 361
Tibial tendons 54
Tibialis posterior tendon 121, 366
Tibiocalcaneal ligament 209
Tibiofibular joint 22, 271
Tibiofibular syndesmosis 365, 366
Tibioperoneal trunk 331, 332, 361
Tibiotalar ligament 209
Toe(s) 26, 59, 120, 392
Tongue muscles 56, 148, 276, 392
Tonsils, palatine 117
Torcular herophili 210
Trachea 90, 114, 149, 216, 239, 364
    carina 52, 395, 453
    double aortic arch 274–5
    persistent left SVC 303
    'retro' spaces 306
    thyroid gland 427
Transverse cervical artery 210
Transverse colon 24, 82, 83, 85, 122,
    243

Transverse ligament 29
Transverse sinuses 24, 210
Transversus abdominis muscle 244,
    452, 453
Trapezium bone 114, 360
Trapezius muscle 240, 272, 273, 276,
    305
Trapezoid bone 114
Treitz, ligament of 176
Triangular fibrocartilage complex 360
Triceps brachii tendon 453
Tricuspid valve 27, 54, 423
Trigeminal nerve (CN V) 89, 151, 302
Trigone, retromolar 180
Triquetral bone 114, 337
Triradiate cartilage 152, 215, 453
Trochanter
    greater 59, 146, 215, 245, 397, 421
    lesser 55, 91, 146, 179, 421
Trochlea 29, 119, 120, 183, 273, 302,
    330, 453
Tuberculum sellae 451
Tunica albuginea 181
Tunica vaginalis 181
Turbinates (conchae), nasal 425
Tympanic cavity (middle ear) 246
Tympanic membrane 245, 246

U
Ulna
    collateral arteries 214
    coronoid process 238, 302, 453,
    454
    distal 150
    key structures of forearm 450
    olecranon 29, 119, 330, 426, 453–4
    radio-ulnar joint 114
    sagittal MRI of elbow 453–4
    styloid process 82, 114
Ulnar artery 214, 307
Ulnar nerve 307
Umbilical arteries 336, 337
    catheters 274
Umbilical cord 336, 337
Umbilical fold, median 277
Umbilical veins 92, 336, 337
    catheters 274
Uncinate process 176, 300
Uncovertebral joint 300
Ureters 87, 396
Urethra 24–5, 179, 241, 331, 396
Urethrography, retrograde 25
Urinary bladder 59, 115, 179, 210, 240,
    268, 338
    maternal 456
    micturating cystourethrography
    396
    transabdominal ultrasound 393
Urinary tract infections 396
Urography 53, 87
Uterine artery 213, 214, 393
Uterus 58, 115, 116, 210, 211, 239,
    268–9,
    301, 393

V
Vagina 115, 268, 269
Vagus nerve (CN X) 28, 209
Valleculae 364
Valsalva, sinuses of 88, 151
Varicocoeles 23, 181
Vas deferens 455
Vastus intermedius muscle 184, 364
Vastus lateralis muscle 115, 364
Vastus medialis muscle 364
Vena cava
    anatomical levels 242
    embryological development 92
    inferior see Inferior vena cava (IVC)
    superior 26, 91, 92, 144, 177, 303,
    365, 425
Venography, pulmonary 54
Venous sinuses, confluence of 210
Ventricles, cardiac
    apical four-chamber echocardio-
    gram 148
    axial imaging 211–12
    heart border silhouette 146, 395
    identification 332
    identifying left/right side of thorax
    and 22
    interventricular septum 27, 56,
    148, 211, 332
    left 451
    oblique coronal view 243
    papillary muscles 56, 243, 268, 423
    pulmonary trunk 54, 330
    'retro' spaces 306
    right coronary artery 88
    sagittal views 149
    septal defects 27, 332
    systemic venous drainage 91
Ventricles, cerebral 27, 52, 115, 119, 181
    cerebellum and CSF spaces 181, 182
    coronal images 304
    motor cortex 390
    neonates 214, 365
    on view of oculomotor nerve 269
Vertebral arteries 23, 26, 58, 146, 210,
    241, 242, 246, 455, 456
    brachial plexus and 304, 305
    common variations 391
    coursing superiorly 361
    MR angiogram 364
    on view of oculomotor nerve 269
Vertebral bodies
    articulation of ribs 300
    L4 26
    L5 331, 336
    posterior longitudinal ligament 29
    T10 242
Vertebrobasilar circulation 146–7,
    241–2, 246, 361
Verumontanum 241
Vesicoureteric reflux 396
Vestibular nerves 151, 213
Vestibule, inner ear 145, 151
Vestibulocochlear nerve (CN VIII) 52,
    53, 151, 213
Vitelline duct 92
Vitreous humour 335

Vocal cords 183–4, 427
Vomer 275

W

Water's projection 333
Wharton, duct of 270
White matter tracts 420

Winking owl sign 118
Wormian bone 307, 421
Wrist 82, 114, 216, 238, 268
    carpal tunnel 307
    mnemonic for carpal bones 360
    ossification centres 337
    tendons 150

X

Xiphoid process (xiphisternum) 116

Z

Zygoma 333
Zygomatic arch 28, 243